OSCEsmart

50 Medical Student OSCEs
in General Practice

Dr. Nisha A. Patel

Executive Consulting Editor:
Dr. Sam Thenabadu

Ordering Information: Quantity sales. Special discounts are available on quantity purchases by corporations, associations, and others. For details, contact the publisher at the address above.

Orders by UK trade bookstores and wholesalers please visit www.scowenpublishing.com

Although every effort has been made to check this text, it is possible that errors have been made, readers are urged to check with the most up to date guidelines and safety regulations.

The authors and the publishers do not accept responsibility or legal liability for any errors in the text, or for the misuse of the material in this book.

Publisher's Cataloging-in-Publication data : OSCEsmart 50 medical student OSCEs in General Practice.

Copyright © 2017 Simon Cowen Publishing

ISBN-10: 0-9908538-9-6
ISBN-13: 978-0-9908538-9-3

CONTENTS

Message from the authors

Doctors of all seniorities can remember the stress of the OSCE but even more so the stress of trying to study and practice for the OSCEs. A multitude of generic undergraduate and postgraduate resources can be found on line but quality, quantity, and completeness of content can vary. The aim of the OSCESmart editorial team is to bring together specialty focused books that have identified 50 core stations encompassing the essential categories of history taking, examinations, emergency moulages, clinical skills and data interpretation with a strong theme of communications running through all the stations.

The combined experience of consultants, registrars and junior doctors to write, edit and quality check these stations, promises to deliver content that is appropriate to reach a standard we would expect of new junior doctors entering their foundation internship years and into core training. It is important to know that these stations are all newly written and based at the level of clinical competencies we would expect from these grades of doctors. Learning objectives exist for undergraduate curricula and for the foundation years, and the scenarios are based and written around these. What they are not, are scenarios that have been 'borrowed' from any medical school.

Preparation is the key to success in most things, but never more so than for the OSCEs and a candidate that hasn't practised will soon be found out. These books will allow you to practice relevant scenarios with verified checklists to learn both content and the generic approach. The format will allow you to practice in groups with one person being the candidate, one the actor and one the examiner. Each scenario finishes with three learning points. Picture these as are three core learning tips that we would want you to take away if you had only a couple of days left to the exam. These OSCE scenarios promise to be a robust revision aide for the student looking to recap and consolidate for their exams, but equally importantly prepare them for life in clinical practice.

I am immensely proud of this OSCESmart series. I have had the pleasure of working with some of the brightest and most dynamic young clinicians and educators I know, and I am sure you will find this series covering the essential clinical specialties a truly robust and invaluable companion in those stressful times of revision. I must take this opportunity to thank my colleagues for all their hard work but most of all to thank my wonderful wife Molly for her unerring love and support and my sons Reuben and Rafael for all the joy they bring me.

Despite the challenging times the health service finds itself in, being a doctor remains a huge privilege. We hope that this OSCESmart series goes some way to help you achieve the excellence you and your patients deserve.

Best of luck, Dr Sam Thenabadu

Introduction to OSCESmart 50 OSCES in General Practice:

I am delighted and privileged to be able to write the foreword for this amazing book on OSCE exams in a general practice setting. The emphasis on general practice osce stations has increased over the past few years, and will continue to do so as changes are made to the medical school curriculum and of course to the NHS.

This book is designed to guide you and give you the essential skills you need to take a thorough but focussed history and in some cases the examination, followed by investigations and management. I have covered a wide range of common topics that come up in exams but also will help in your future career. Unlike the other books in the series I have split the chapters into specialities, and within each chapter are topics that can be fairly difficult to deal with in a general practice environment, therefore prompt appropriate follow up or management plans.

There is an art to general practice which is centered around 'ideas, concerns and expectations' and of course excellent communication skills. You will notice many of the mark schemes have a specific section for addressing ICE, and for recognising non verbal and verbal cues. Additionally I have included a chapter on communication skills, mainly to highlight the importance of building a rapport with your patients and emphasizing its importance in maintaining good clinical practice.

I would like to take this opportunity to thank my grandparents whose faith in my abilities has given me strength to continually fulfil my potential. I would like to give a special mention to my brother, Kishan who never fails to make me laugh and has been patient enough to take my photo multiple times for this book, until it was perfect. Lastly, my accomplishments to date would not have been achieved without the sacrifices made by my Dad and Mum, who have guided and supported me throughout my life, for which I am and always will be eternally grateful.

I would also like to say a big thank you to all my co-authors for their commitment to this project and their patience with my endless emails and pestering. Without them this book would not have been possible. In addition I would like to express my gratitude to Dr Sam Thenabadu, who gave me this amazing opportunity and has been a great mentor over the past year.

I hope you will find this book useful in your exam preparation. Good luck to you all with your exams and also your future career!

Nisha Patel

About the Authors

Dr Nisha Patel

MBBS BSc (Hons)

ST1 Paediatrics

Dr Nisha Patel graduated from Imperial College, London in 2014 with a Distinction in Surgery, Obstetrics and Gynaecology and Merit in Medicine. She also graduated with a 2:1 for her Reproductive and Developmental Sciences BSc. She completed her foundation training at St Richard's Hospital, Chichester and Princess Royal University Hospital, Kent, where she was awarded a Certificate of Merit for her Learning Portfolio and Certificate of Merit for Leadership, respectively.

She has an interest in Clinical Audit and Quality Improvement projects, with both oral and poster presentations at international and national conferences. Dr Patel has promoted team building and morale within the multidisciplinary team, by taking on leadership roles including Mess President, Social Secretary and currently Rota Coordinator. She recognises the importance of teaching and helping with preparation for clinical exams, therefore organises an annual Paediatric PACES course for Imperial College students. She runs workshops at the Imperial Paediatrics Conference focussing on patient-centered consultations and communication skills.

Her biggest achievement is her commitment to the Paediatrics Society at Imperial College, which she founded in 2012. The society's main project is the Student Play Team, where Dr Patel facilitated a group of over 150 volunteers who dedicate their evenings and weekends to play with children on the wards, at St Mary's Hospital, Paddington. The aim was to maximise on students' energy and drive to engage children in hospital and improve patient experience whilst providing learning opportunities for students in child interaction and teamwork.

She is currently a Paediatric trainee in the London School of Paediatrics at Queen Elizabeth Hospital, Woolwich.

Dr Sam Thenabadu

MBBS MRCP DRCOG DCH MA Clin Ed FRCEM MSc (Paed) FHEA

Consultant Adult & Paediatric Emergency Medicine
Honorary Senior Lecturer & Associate Director of Medical Education

Sam Thenabadu graduated from King's College Medical School in 2001 and dual trained in Adult and Paediatric Emergency Medicine in London before being appointed a consultant in 2011 at the Princess Royal University Hospital. He has Masters degrees in Clinical Medical Education and Advanced Paediatrics.

He is undergraduate director of medical education at the King's College NHS Trust and the academic block lead for Emergency Medicine and Critical Care at King's College School of Medicine. At postgraduate level he has been the Pan London Health Education England lead for CT3 paediatric emergency medicine trainees since 2011. Academically he has previously written two textbooks and has published in peer review journals and given numerous oral and poster presentations at national conferences in emergency medicine, paediatrics, medical education and patient quality and safety.

He has an unashamed passion for medical education and strives to achieve excellence for himself, his colleagues and his patients, hoping to always deliver this through an enjoyable learning environment. Service delivery and educational need not be two separate entities, and he hopes that those who have had great teachers will take it upon themselves to do the same for others in the future.

Co- Authors

Dr Dugald Brown Bsc, MBBS

Dr Yee-Teng Chon Bsc (Hons), MBBS

Dr Malaz Elsaddig Bsc MBBS
Clinical Teaching Fellow, University of Bristol, Swindon Academy at Great Western Hospital

Dr Rhiannon Jones MBBS, MA (Cantab)
Emergency Department, Senior Resident Medical Officer, Australia

Dr Balrik Kailey MBBS, BA
Core Medical Trainee, London

Dr Vishal Kumar MBBS
Cardio-Respiratory CT1, Leicester

Dr Kristina Nanthagopan Bsc (Hons), MBBS
GPST2, London

Dr Christiana Page MBChB
Intensive Care Clinical Fellow, London

Dr Naim Slim Bsc MBBS
Anatomy Demonstrator & Junior Clinical Fellow (General Surgery), University of Cambridge

Chapter 1: Cardiology

Case 1: Shortness of Breath

Candidate's Instructions

You are the foundation year doctor working in General Practice and have been asked to see a 65 year old lady, Anna who presents to your practice complaining of shortness of breath. She is clinically stable.

After 6 minutes the examiner will stop you and ask you to summarise back your findings, suggest your differential diagnoses and your initial management plan.

Examiner's Instructions

A 65 year old lady Anna, presents to the general practice complaining of shortness of breath. She is clinically stable.

The candidate, is acting as the foundation year doctor, and has been asked to take a history from the patient.

After 6 minutes please stop the candidate at whatever stage they are and ask them to present the case with their primary differential diagnoses. Following this ask them what their next steps regarding investigations and management will be.

If they ask, give them the examination findings below:
Examination findings: Mrs Langley is short of breath after walking down the long corridor to your consultation room. Her obs are stable. On examination her jugular venous pressure is raised at 2cm, heart sounds are normal, chest is clear, abdomen shows no evidence of organomegaly. She has bilateral pitting oedema to the level of the ankle.
Questions to ask if there is time:
What changes would you expect to see on a chest xray showing heart failure?
What medications are given to heart failure patients?

Actor's Instructions

You are a 65 year old lady Anna, who has attended the general practice with shortness of breath that has been getting steadily worse over the past 2 months.

ONLY OFFER INFORMATION IF SPECIFICALLY ASKED

You previously used to be able to walk up a hill without too much trouble but now walking 20m on a flat down to the shops is making you short of breath.

You have a mild cough (2 weeks) with occasionally bringing up white sputum. There is no blood or green phlegm.

You are finding it more difficult to sleep at night finding some relief with three pillows.

You have noticed some ankle swelling on both sides. There is no redness and it is equal on both sides.

You have noticed no weight loss, change in appetite or night sweats.

You have no dizziness, chest pain, palpitations or fever.

You have no history of clots or recent travel.

You have previously suffered a heart attack 5 years ago and have high cholesterol and diabetes. You are on Bisoprolol, Ramipril, Simvastatin, Metformin and Gliclazide. You have no drug allergies.

You are a smoker (20 a day for 50 years) and drink the occasional glass of red wine. You used to be a receptionist.

You have no relevant family history.

If asked about your ideas, concerns and expectations please offer the information below

You are concerned this may be cancer as you have heard on the news breathlessness can be a sign of lung cancer and with your history of smoking you are 100% this is the diagnosis.

Mark Scheme: Shortness of Breath

Task:	Achieved	Not Achieved
Introduces himself / herself		
Confirms patient details and purpose of consultation		
Established the main presenting complaint and elicits progressive nature of shortness of breath		
Explores symptom of worsening shortness of breath (duration, onset (sudden / gradual), timing, exacerbating and relieving factors, exercise tolerance) and compares to baseline		
Explores symptom of cough (duration, whether cough is productive, coryzal symptoms) and compares to baseline		
Elicits ankle swelling		
Elicits SOB worse when lying flat and number of pillows needed for comfort.		
Asks about chest pain and syncope		
Asks about pulmonary embolism risk factors - previous clots, recent surgery, recent travel.		
Asks about red flags – weight loss, change in appetite, haemoptysis, night sweats		
Asks about past medical history specifically previous cardiac history		
Asks about medications and allergies		
Asks about family history & social history including occupation, alcohol and smoking		
Plans to examine or asks for examination findings		

Summarises findings concisely		
Able to provide appropriate differential diagnoses Heart Failure Acute Non Infective Exacerbation of COPD Pulmonary Embolism Lung Cancer		
Suggests appropriate investigations Routine Bloods - FBC- to exclude anaemia, BNP - measure of heart failure. ECG and Chest xray May require ECHO to assess Left ventricular function		
Appropriate management plan & follow-up Lifestyle changes Start medications including Follow up in 2 weeks to review.		
Acknowledges & addresses patient's ideas, concerns and expectations		
Gives patient opportunity to ask questions		
Examiner's Global Mark	/5	
Actor / Helper's Global Mark	/5	
Total Station Mark	/30	

Learning Points

- Know the constellation of associated symptoms that present with each differential for shortness of breath. Eg: infectious symptoms for chest infection, triggers and pleuritic pain for PE and peripheral oedema, orthopnoea and cardiac history for heart failure.

- Think about risk factors and what the patient's main concern may be early so you can prepare for it and ensure you can reassure them. Sometimes you may not know the answer to their questions, in this case tell the truth, and offer them an additional resource, leaflet or find out for them and inform them at a follow up appointment.

- Initial management of heart failure is important that you will see throughout your career, learn the first line medications and their mechanism of actions for both primary and secondary care. NICE guidelines exist to provide a framework for investigation and management.

Case 2: Chest Pain

Candidate's Instructions

You are the foundation year doctor working in General Practice and have been asked to see a 65 year old gentleman Anthony who presents to your practice complaining of chest discomfort.

After 6 minutes the examiner will stop you and ask you to summarise back your findings, suggest your differential diagnoses and your initial management plan.

Examiner's Instructions

The candidate, is acting as the foundation year doctor, and has been asked to take a history from Anthony a 65 year old gentleman who presents to the general practice complaining of chest discomfort.

Please note as the patient gives a history of a patient with acute coronary syndrome, the candidate may stop and say that they would manage the patient using the Airway, breathing, circulation assessment. Just guide them to continue the history at this point.

After 6 minutes please stop the candidate at whatever stage they are and ask them to present the case with their primary differential diagnoses. Following this ask them what their next steps regarding investigations and management will be.

If they ask, give them the examination findings below:
Examination findings:
A: Airway patent.
B: Chest clear, equal air entry bilaterally. Respiratory Rate 35 and saturations 92% on air.
C: Heart rate 120, regular and blood pressure stable at 135/86. You do not have an ECG machine.
D: GCS 15/15, Blood glucose 8.9, normal neurology. Temperature 37degrees.
E: Abdomen soft and non tender, no other signs of acute illness.
Questions to ask if there is time:
What medication would you have in stock at a General Practice that you could give in the interim if suspecting Acute Coronary Syndrome? What dose?

Actor's Instructions

You are a 65 year old gentleman Anthony, who has attended the GP with chest discomfort that started this morning while you were walking to the train station 30 minutes ago.

ONLY OFFER INFORMATION IF SPECIFICALLY ASKED

The chest pain is central and dull in nature, severity 6/10. It is constant in nature (does not come and go). The pain travels up to your jaw but not through to your back. The chest pain is still currently present during the consultation. Nothing is making it better or worse, you did try taking some paracetamol while in the waiting room. Specifically the pain is not worse with breathing, but you are very short of breath. You are sweaty and very anxious. You have no dizziness/cough/fever. You have also been feeling nauseous but have not vomited yet.

This is the first time you have had chest pain like this. You can normally walk and exercise without chest pain. However you do not exercise very much, apart from walking to and from the train station.

Your past medical history includes hypertension, diabetes and high cholesterol. You have no previous cardiac history. You are on Ramipril, Simvastatin and Metformin. You have no drug allergies.

You have no calf swelling or tenderness. You have not been on a recent long haul flight, or had recent surgery, and you have not had a previous clot before.

You are a smoker (20 a day for 50 years) and drink 5 pints of beer a week. You take no recreational drugs. You are a teacher.

Your mother died from a clot in her lungs a few years ago.

If asked about your ideas, concerns and expectations please offer the information below

You are concerned this may be a clot on the lungs (like your mother) and are worried you will also die, you would have gone to the emergency department but you were closer to your GP surgery. You ask if you are going to send him to ED.

Case 2: Chest Pain

Task:	Achieved	Not Achieved
Introduces himself / herself		
Confirms patient details and purpose of consultation		
Established the main presenting complaint and if he has previously had episodes of this nature		
Ascertains site of pain and radiation		
Elicits timing, onset and character of pain		
Asks specifically about radiation through to back, neck and arm		
Asks about associated symptoms: shortness of breath, nausea and sweating		
Elicits that pain is not pleuritic, and there is no calf swelling or pain.		
Asks about risks factors for pulmonary embolism - recent long haul flight, surgery, previous history of clot		
Asks about past medical history specifically previous cardiac risk factors - diabetes, hypertension and high cholesterol		
Asks about medications and allergies		
Asks about family history & social history including alcohol and smoking		
Plans to examine or asks for examination findings - may ask to stabilise patient first before continuing with history.		
Calls for help early		

Summarises findings concisely		
Able to provide appropriate differential diagnoses Acute Coronary Syndrome Pulmonary Embolism Atypical presentation of dissection		
Suggests appropriate investigations Urgent set of observations ECG		
Appropriate management plan & follow-up To call ambulance for a blue light ?ACS To give patient Oxygen and attach monitoring To regularly review patient while waiting for ambulance To give GTN spray and aspirin		
Acknowledges & addresses patient's ideas, concerns and expectations		
Gives patient opportunity to ask questions		
Examiner's Global Mark	/5	
Actor / Helper's Global Mark	/5	
Total Station Mark	/30	

Learning Points

- Know the important features of the classical history for a presentation of acute coronary syndrome. It is important to identify the nuances of the features of chest pain to help point you towards acute coronary syndrome, pulmonary embolism, aortic dissection and then the less serious differentials.

- Knowing when to call for help is crucial. Even in a General Practice, patients like this can walk through the doors. Remember there are nursing staff and senior practitioners who may be able to help. Calling an ambulance to a GP practice is more than acceptable if the patient urgently requires hospitalisation.

- General practices have a stock of medication including oxygen, aspirin, GTN spray and other medications that are for emergency use, they also have a defibrillator in case of emergencies.

Case 3: Collapse

Candidate's Instructions

You are the foundation year doctor working in General Practice and have been asked to see James a 70 year old gentleman who presents to your practice following a collapse.

After 6 minutes the examiner will stop you and ask you to summarise back your findings, suggest your differential diagnoses and your initial management plan.

Examiner's Instructions

Mr Jone, a 70 year old gentleman presents to the general practice complaining of an episode of collapse.

The candidate, is acting as the foundation year doctor, and has been asked to take a history from the patient.

After 6 minutes please stop the candidate at whatever stage they are and ask them to present the case with their primary differential diagnoses. Following this ask them what their next steps regarding investigations and management will be. T

If they ask, give them the examination findings below:
Examination findings: Mr Jones is sat comfortably at rest. His observations are within the normal range. Cardiovascular examination reveals an ejection systolic murmur, heard loudest in the right 2nd intercostal space which radiates to the carotids. All other systemic examinations are normal.
Questions to ask if there is time:
What is the difference between aortic stenosis and aortic sclerosis?
What surgical treatment could be provided for aortic stenosis?

Actor's Instructions

You are a 70 year old gentleman James, who has attended the GP following a collapse over the weekend.

ONLY OFFER INFORMATION IF SPECIFICALLY ASKED

You collapsed whilst going for a brisk walk. You felt worsening 'light-headedness' in the minute prior to the fall. You fainted and fell to the ground but did not lose consciousness. Everything went out of focus but the landscape was not spinning around you

You were not incontinent, nor did you have any seizures. You did not notice any preceding palpitations. You find that you do get chest tightness again on exertion.

You were also quite short of breath but had not noticed any other symptoms. You have found that you are getting progressing shortness of breath. Now you can only walk 100 yards on a flat before getting short of breath whereas previously you could walk a mile on a slight incline.

Your wife witnessed the whole event and can attest there was no seizure/incontinence.

You have suffered similar episodes before (not as severe) and they tend to occur when you are exercising.

Your past medical history includes hypertension, diabetes and high cholesterol. You have no previous cardiac history. You are on Ramipril, Simvastatin and Metformin. No drug allergies.

You are a smoker (20 a day for 50 years) and drink 5 pints of beer a week. You take no recreational drugs. You used to work in a bank, but are now retired.

Your mother passed away following a stroke aged 80.

If asked about your ideas, concerns and expectations please offer the information below

You are concerned the next time this happens you might black out completely with no-one else around.

Mark Scheme: Collapse

Task:	Achieved	Not Achieved
Introduces himself / herself		
Confirms patient details and purpose of consultation		
Established the main presenting complaint and elicits circumstances of collapse		
Elicits pre-syncopal symptoms and palpitations		
Elicits no LOC/seizure/incontinence		
Elicits lack of vertiginous symptoms.		
Asks about witnesses		
Elicits previous history of exertional pre-syncope		
Elicits progressively worsening SOB on exertion		
Elicits symptoms of exertional (stable) angina.		
Asks about past medical history specifically previous cardiac history		
Asks about medications and allergies		
Asks about family history & social history including alcohol and smoking		
Summarises findings concisely		
Plans to examine or asks for examination findings		
Able to provide appropriate differential diagnoses Aortic stenosis Arrhythmia Vasovagal syncope		
Suggests appropriate investigations Basic Bloods - FBC - exclude anaemia CXR and ECG ECHO		
Appropriate management plan & follow-up Follow up with blood test results and imaging Optimise medication for other risk factors e.g. blood pressure control, diabetes & cholesterol		

May require cardiology referral depending on the results of investigations.		
Acknowledges & addresses patient's ideas, concerns and expectations		
Gives patient opportunity to ask questions		
Examiner's Global Mark	/5	
Actor / Helper's Global Mark	/5	
Total Station Mark	/30	

Learning Points

- When taking a history of collapse it is crucial to ascertain if there was definite loss of consciousness and whether there were any witnesses.

- It is important to be able to differentiate between pre-syncopal symptoms and true vertigo when patients complain of 'feeling dizzy'. In order to achieve this asking open questions can allow patients to describe the event in more details allowing a better understanding of the symptoms.

- The triad of exertional SOB, angina and exertional syncope is classical of symptomatic aortic stenosis. The latter is a late sign suggestive of disease severe enough to cause cerebral hypoperfusion.

Case 4: Palpitations

Candidate's Instructions

You are the foundation year doctor working in General Practice and have been asked to see Amanda a 50 year old lady who presents to your practice after experiencing palpitations.

After 6 minutes the examiner will stop you and ask you to summarise back your findings, suggest your differential diagnoses and your initial management plan.

Examiner's Instructions

Amanda a 50 year old lady presents to the General Practice complaining of palpitations.

The candidate, is acting as the foundation year doctor, and has been asked to take a history from the patient.

After 6 minutes please stop the candidate at whatever stage they are and ask them to present the case with their primary differential diagnoses. Following this ask them what their next steps regarding investigations and management will be.

If they ask, give them the examination findings below:
Examination findings: Mrs Adams is comfortable at rest and does not look like she is in any discomfort. Her observations are within normal ranges. However on palpation of her pulse, it feels irregularly irregular. All other systemic examinations are normal.
Questions to ask if there is time:
What are the common causes of Atrial Fibrillation?
What is the CHA_2DS_2VAS Score?

Actor's Instructions

You are a 50 year old lady Amanda, who has come to the GP as you are worried about the palpitations you have been having recently.

ONLY OFFER INFORMATION IF SPECIFICALLY ASKED
It feels uncomfortable because you become very aware of your own heartbeat and it seems really fast. They last about a few minutes and tend to disappear when you rest. They first started a year ago and seem to be getting worse. They come on often when you exercising and occasionally at rest. There is no prior warning.

There is occasional central chest tightness. This is a non-radiating, dull pain, 4/10 in severity and disappears as the palpitations do.

There is no shortness of breath or feeling faint.

You haven't noticed any weight loss or change in appetite. You dress appropriately for the weather and you do not sweat over much.
You do not suffer from headaches.

You have no other medical problems and are not on any medications and have no allergies.

You are a smoker (10 a day for 20 years) and drink in binges. You have the occasional coffee. You take no recreational drugs. You are a lawyer.

Your mother passed away of breast cancer when she was 65.

If asked about your ideas, concerns and expectations please offer the information below

You are concerned that these episodes will one day lead to a heart attack and you will die early.

Mark Scheme: Collapse

Task:	Achieved	Not Achieved
Introduces himself / herself		
Confirms patient details and purpose of consultation		
Established the main presenting complaint		
Elicits palpitations and their length and pattern		
Elicits lack of prior warning		
Elicits associated chest pain & shortness of breath		
Asks about pre-syncopal symptoms		
Asks about thyroid related symptoms: sweating and temperature control, weight changes		
Asks about headache.		
Asks about social history including caffeine, alcohol & smoking		
Asks about past medical history		
Asks about medications and allergies		
Asks about family history		
Plans to examine or asks for examination findings		
Summarises findings concisely		
Able to provide appropriate differential diagnoses Atrial Fibrillation Sinus Tachycardia - ?anxiety related or normal variant Other arrhythmia		
Suggests appropriate investigations Basic Bloods: FBC - to exclude anaemia, TFTs - to exclude thyroid related atrial fibrillation ECG 24hr tape or 7day monitor		
Appropriate management plan & follow-up Follow up after the investigations Consider alternative causes e.g. Hyperthyroidism Consider medical treatment using rhythm control as <65yrs		

Consider anticoagulation using the CHA2DS2VAS Score Seek expert advice		
Acknowledges & addresses patient's ideas, concerns and expectations		
Gives patient opportunity to ask questions		
Examiner's Global Mark	/5	
Actor / Helper's Global Mark	/5	
Total Station Mark	/30	

Learning Points

- Palpitations are a common complaint in general practice and it is important to realize how concerning they can be for the patient. Therefore you must take into consideration the impact these symptoms are having on activities of daily living.

- It is important to think about the likely causes in different groups of patients i.e age, thryrotoxicosis, alcohol, caffeine and recreational drugs

- A normal ECG does not preclude AF/arrhythmia and if the palpitations are occasional longer monitoring should be considered to help pick any underlying rhythm.

Case 5: Hypertension Management

Candidate's Instructions

You are the foundation year doctor working in General Practice. The practice nurse has asked this 60 year old gentleman Peter to see you as his blood pressure was 150/95 mmHg on three separate occasions last week.

After 6 minutes the examiner will stop you and ask you to summarise back your findings, suggest your differential diagnoses and your initial management plan.

Examiner's Instructions:

A 60 year old gentleman, Peter, has been asked to see a doctor as the practice nurse noticed his blood pressure was elevated.

The candidate, is acting as the foundation year doctor Doctor, and has been asked to take a brief history from the patient.

After 6 minutes, please stop the candidate and ask:

"Please summarise your findings and discuss how you would like to investigate and manage this patient."

If they ask, give them the examination findings below:
Examination findings: Mr Pritchard is well, but overweight. His weight today is 93kg. His BMI is 30. You specifically measure his blood pressure, the best of three readings was 152/92.
Questions to ask if there is time:
What is the first-line treatment you would initiate if hypertension was confirmed?
What would you consider if this didn't work?

Actor's Instructions:

You are a 60 year old gentleman Peter, who has recently signed up at the GP practice. You visited the practice nurse who noticed your blood pressure was high and has asked you to see the doctor.

ONLY OFFER INFORMATION IF SPECIFICALLY ASKED
You have had no obvious symptoms. You feel well in yourself.

You have Type 2 Diabetes for which you are on Metformin and have no allergies.

Your father died of a heart attack aged 60.

You have smoked 20 cigarettes a day for 40 years. You drink a couple pints every weekend.

Your diet consists of a 'fry-up' in the morning, some sandwiches for lunch and often a takeaway for dinner. You snack often. You have quite a lot of salt in your diet. You have been gaining weight slowly over the past few years and now weigh 90kg.

You rarely exercise, but you are a builder and your work consists of manual labour and therefore feel it is enough.

The candidate will now have a discussion with the examiner. Following this they will take some time to address your ideas, concerns and expectations. You have some specific questions:

1. What does high blood pressure mean?
2. Your father had high blood pressure and he died of a heart attack will the same happen to you?
3. What food should you avoid?
4. Which medications will they start for high blood pressure and what are the side effects?

Mark Scheme: Hypertension management

Task:	Achieved	Not Achieved
Introduces himself / herself		
Confirms patient details and purpose of consultation		
Takes a brief history, establishing lack of symptoms.		
Asks about past medical history- asking specifically about cardiac history, diabetes, high cholesterol.		
Asks about medications and allergies		
Asks about family history & social history including alcohol and smoking		
Elicits other risk factors - diet, exercise, weight gain.		
Summarises findings concisely		
Able to identify that this patient may have Hypertension		
Plans to examine or asks for examination findings		
Suggests appropriate investigations Blood tests - cholesterol, HbA1c, renal function Urine dip - assess for end organ damage		
Appropriate management plan & follow-up Monitor blood pressure at home Initiates antihypertensive according to guidelines Follow up in 2 weeks with blood pressure diary		
Explains probable diagnosis is hypertension and explains what this in lay terms for patient.		
Explains need for ambulatory blood pressure monitoring to confirm diagnosis.		
Discusses need for low salt-diet and change to exercise regime		
Discusses smoking cessation		
Offers at least one resource or community intervention.		
Discusses possibly needing to start medication and explains the side effects		
Acknowledges & addresses patient's ideas, concerns and expectations		

Gives patient opportunity to ask questions		
Examiner's Global Mark	/5	
Actor / Helper's Global Mark	/5	
Total Station Mark	/30	

Learning Points

- It is important to always start with lifestyle interventions to help the patient take ownership of their disease. Offer them different community resources and interventions to help e.g. smoking cessation nurses, dieticians and group exercise classes.

- With a new diagnosis of hypertension it is important to think of other cardiovascular risk factors and how to assess for end-organ damage.

- With management stations spend less time on the history and focus on a simple explanation of the diagnosis and the upcoming management rationale.

Chapter 2: Respiratory

Case 1: Chronic Obstructive Pulmonary Disease

Candidate Instructions

You are the foundation year doctor working in General Practice and have been asked to see a 70 year old woman Diana, who has presented to the GP surgery complaining of increased breathlessness and cough.

After 6 minutes the examiner will stop you and ask you to summarise back your findings, suggest your differential diagnoses and your initial management plan.

Examiner Instructions

A 70 year old woman Diana, has presented to the GP surgery complaining of increased breathlessness and cough.

The candidate, is acting as the foundation year doctor Doctor, and has been asked to take a history from the patient.

After 6 minutes please stop the candidate at whatever stage they are and ask them to present the case with their primary differential diagnoses. Following this ask them what their next steps regarding investigations and management will be.

If the candidate asks the patient to demonstrate inhaler technique inform them that the patient's technique is adequate.

If they ask, give them the examination findings below:
Examination findings: Observations stable, afebrile, saturations 92% on air. The patient is mildly dyspnoeic but there is no visible cyanosis. There is air entry on both sides of the chest with widespread wheeze on auscultation. All other systemic examinations are normal.

Questions to ask if there is time:
- What would the spirometry results of a patient with COPD show?
- What other primary care interventions could improve the control of the COPD?

Actor Instructions

You are a 70 year old woman Diana, who has come to see the GP because you have been feeling more breathless and coughing more than usual in the past week or so.

ONLY OFFER INFORMATION IF SPECIFICALLY ASKED

Normally, you walk slowly and your breathing is not affected, but you get quite breathless going up stairs or hills. You cough early in the morning, often bringing up some white or clear phlegm.

For the past week you have been struggling to walk 100 meters, you have to stop due to your breathing and you have noticed a wheeze. You have been using your blue inhaler twice as often as usual. It has been a struggle to continue your everyday activities. During the day you have been coughing more but still bringing up white or clear mucus, no blood.

You have not had fevers or night sweats. You have not lost any weight recently.

You do not struggle with breathing when lying flat and you do not wake suddenly from sleep very short of breath.

You have had no pain or swelling in your legs. No recent foreign travel or long-haul flights and no recent contact with anyone with an infection.

You have COPD (diagnosed 10 years ago). You have had fairly frequent chest infections (2-3 per year) but you have only been admitted to hospital 2-3 times in total. You have never needed intensive care. You have no known heart problems and no history of previous clots

You take Seretide one puff twice a day, Spiriva one puff once a day, your blue salbutamol inhaler as and when you need it. You have been taking your medication as prescribed.

You had trouble with inhaler technique so you now use a spacer and have no problems with it. You do not have home oxygen or home nebulisers. You have the flu vaccine every year. You have no allergies.

You have a family history of high blood pressure. You are not aware of any lung cancer in the family. You were a secondary school teacher but retired 5 years ago. You live with your husband and you are both still independent and physically active. You are an ex-smoker (20 a day for 40 years) and you quit about 10 years ago. You do not drink. You do not have any pets.

If asked about your ideas, concerns and expectations please offer the information below
You're not sure what is causing your symptoms. When your symptoms have got worse like this in the past it is usually due to a chest infection. You are concerned that this is not just a transient worsening of your symptoms but the disease progressing.

Mark Scheme: Chronic Obstructive Pulmonary Disease

Task:	Achieved	Not Achieved
Introduces himself / herself		
Confirms patient details and purpose of consultation		
Established the main presenting complaint		
Explores symptom of worsened breathlessness - duration, onset (sudden / gradual), timing, exacerbating and relieving factors, exercise tolerance, use of inhalers- and compares to baseline		
Explores symptom of cough - duration, whether cough is productive, coryzal symptoms - and compares to baseline		
Asks about red flags – weight loss, change in appetite, haemoptysis, night sweats		
Asks about chest pain and leg swelling		
Asks about past medical history specifically previous history of respiratory and cardiac disease and venous thrombo-embolism		
Establishes history of COPD - age at diagnosis, nature of symptoms, admissions to hospital / intensive care		
Asks about medications and allergies		
Asks about family history & social history including alcohol and smoking		
Checks inhaler technique (candidate informed that it is adequate)		
Checks adherence to medication (and that medication is in date)		

Plans to examine or asks for examination findings		
Summarises findings concisely		
Able to provide appropriate differential diagnoses Acute Non Infective Exacerbation of COPD Acute infective exacerbation of COPD Heart Failure Pulmonary Embolism Lung Cancer		
Suggests appropriate investigations Blood test Chest x-ray Spirometry to assess worsening COPD Carbon monoxide monitoring		
Appropriate management plan & follow-up 5-7 day course of oral prednisolone Arrange a rescue pack of antibiotics to take away and be used in case infection develops Review in 6 weeks +/- chest x-ray Consider adjunct treatment such as mucolytic, dietary supplements, psychological support Pulmonary rehabilitation		
Acknowledges & addresses patient's ideas, concerns and expectations		
Gives patient opportunity to ask questions		
Examiner's Global Mark	/5	
Actor / Helper's Global Mark	/5	
Total Station Mark	/30	

Learning Points

- Even if you know that a patient has a chronic condition such as COPD from the outset, which in this case you do not, it's important to take the history of the presenting symptoms with an open mind. Not every patient with COPD who comes in with increased shortness of breath is going to have an exacerbation of their COPD. Think about the differential diagnosis systematically.

- When taking a history of breathlessness always establish level of function and compare to *their* baseline. This could be referenced from the distance walked or the activities carried out at home.

- It is important to be aware of the holistic and multidisciplinary care provided in the community for COPD including smoking cessation and pulmonary rehabilitation.

Case 2: Asthma Management

Candidate Instructions

You are a foundation year doctor in the GP surgery who has been asked to see Renata, a 21 year old woman with asthma, who has presented t for her annual asthma review.

After 6 minutes the examiner will stop you and ask you to summarise back your findings, suggest your differential diagnoses and your initial management plan.

Examiner Instructions

Renata a 21 year old woman, has presented to the GP surgery for her annual asthma review.

The candidate, is acting as the foundation year doctor, and has been asked to take a brief history from the patient. After 6 minutes please stop the candidate at whatever stage they are and ask them to present the case and propose their next steps regarding investigations and management.

If they ask, give them the examination findings below:
Examination findings: Renata looks comfortable at rest, observations are stable, chest clear, Peak Expiratory Flow Rate is within the expected range. All other systemic examinations are normal.

Questions to ask if there is time:
What is the next step for asthma management following addition of a long acting beta agonist?
How would you manage a patient with an acute severe exacerbation of their asthma?

Actor Instructions

You are Renata, a 21 year old woman. You have come in for your annual asthma review.

ONLY OFFER INFORMATION IF SPECIFICALLY ASKED
You were diagnosed with asthma when you were 5 years old. Your symptoms worsened in your mid-teens so you were started on a regular brown inhaler. You think the worsening of your symptoms was stress related. Since then your control has been good. You have mild episodes of breathlessness, wheezing and feeling that your chest is tight 3-4 times per year, often triggered by stress at work. On these occasions you use your blue inhaler which rapidly relieves the symptoms.

Symptoms do not routinely interfere with work or exercise and they never wake you from sleep. You have never been admitted to hospital or intensive care due to asthma.

In the past few weeks, however, you have had more frequent symptoms (3-4 times per week). You have used your blue inhaler each time but you are not convinced it works as well as it used to, as symptoms take longer to resolve. You have not had coryzal symptoms, fever or cough.

You are confident that you are using the inhaler properly. You use your brown inhaler every day without fail. You have checked that both your inhalers have doses left in them and that they are within their 'use by dates'.

You have asthma and seasonal hay fever. You have a peak flow meter at home and you think your best was about 420 but you don't measure peak flow regularly.

You don't have a written action plan for your asthma. You take Clenil Modulite 400mcg once a day and Salbutamol 200mcg when required. You take antihistamines when required during pollen season. You have no drug allergies.

You have a family history of asthma and hay fever.

You are a lawyer at a busy firm. You smoked socially in your teens and you have started smoking again, 5-10 cigarettes per day. You do not drink. You live with your long-term boyfriend and you have no pets.

The candidate will now have a discussion with the examiner. Following this they will take some time to address your ideas, concerns and expectations. You have some specific questions:

1. You have been under a lot of stress recently due to a big case at work which is due to come to an end in the next few days. You also understand starting to smoke again will not help the situation. What help could you get with regards to the stress and help with stop smoking?
2. You are concerned that you will need long term steroids and you have read that there are a number of side effects especially if used in high doses, but would like the doctor to explain the side effects.
3. Are there alternative medications instead of just increasing the steroid inhaler?

Mark Scheme: Asthma Management

Task:	Achieved	Not Achieved
Introduces himself / herself		
Confirms patient details and purpose of consultation		
Establishes nature and duration of worsened symptoms of asthma and compare to baseline		
Explores current symptom control: 1) How many times per week do you experience symptoms during the day and how severe are they?		
Explores current symptom control: 2) How many times per week do symptoms wake you from sleep?		
Explores current symptom control: 3) How much do symptoms interfere with usual activities (work / exercise)?		
Explores current symptom control: 4) How many times per week do you use your blue inhaler?		
Checks inhaler technique (candidate informed that it is adequate)		
Checks adherence to medication (and that medication is in date)		
Identifies any trigger factors (airborne irritants e.g. pollen, dust, pets, smoking / weather / infection / acid reflux / exercise / medication / stress)		
Asks about past medical history, medications and allergies, family history & social history including alcohol, occupation and smoking		
Plans to examine or asks for examination findings		
Summarises findings concisely		

Able to identify that this patient has symptoms suggesting poorly controlled asthma		
Appropriate management plan & follow-up Consider changes to medication Smoking cessation nurse referral Follow up and explore stress in more detail Review in 2-3weeks with regards to decision about medication. Suggests creating a written action plan		
Discusses smoking cessation and recent stressors		
Offers at least one resource or community intervention.		
Discusses steroids and explains their side effects and/or alternative medication e.g. LABA		
Acknowledges & addresses patient's ideas, concerns and expectations		
Gives patient opportunity to ask questions		
Examiner's Global Mark	/5	
Actor / Helper's Global Mark	/5	
Total Station Mark	/30	

Learning Points

- It is important to be able to accurately assess the control of asthma symptoms. The questions detailed in the mark scheme are derived from the Royal College of Physicians '3 Questions' and the 'Asthma Control Questionnaire'. You must know the criteria for stepping up on the NICE stepwise protocol for the management of asthma.

- It is important to think holistically about why this patient's control has deteriorated so you can directly address any underlying cause rather than just change medication. Look over the actor's brief and identify all the factors that could influence her control.

- This case is a good example of patient-centred care. We must encourage patients to take ownership of the management of their asthma which is better for the patient and the clinician and hopefully improves adherence. Notice that the mark scheme expects you to *negotiate* a management plan with the patient. To do this you need to give them the information necessary to make an informed decision and you need to understand their concerns and motivations in making that decision.

Case 3: Chronic Cough

Candidate Instructions

You are the foundation year doctor working in General Practice and have been asked to see Jack a 60 year old man who has presented to the GP surgery complaining of a chronic cough.

After 6 minutes the examiner will stop you and ask you to summarise back your findings, suggest yourinvestigations and your initial management plan.

Examiner Instructions

Jack a 60 year old man has presented to the GP surgery with a 2 month history of persistent cough.

The candidate, is acting as the foundation year doctor, and has been asked to take a history from the patient.

After 6 minutes please stop the candidate at whatever stage they are and ask them to present the case with their primary differential diagnoses. Following this ask them what their next steps regarding investigations and management will be.

If they ask, give them the examination findings below:
Examination findings: Mr Jackson looks comfortable at rest, but cachectic, on inspection there is obvious finger clubbing, his chest is clear on auscultation and percussion, normal expansion bilaterally, no lymphadenopathy. All other systemic examinations are normal.

Questions to ask if there is time:
What are the different types of lung cancer? How do they present differently and what is their prognoses?
What are the complications of lung cancer?

Actor Instructions

You are Jack a 60 year old retired missionary. You have had a dry cough for a long time and you have become concerned why it's not going away.
ONLY OFFER INFORMATION IF SPECIFICALLY ASKED
The cough started about 2 months ago and has been present every day since it started. The cough is normally non-productive but you sometimes bring up small amounts of red blood when you cough.

You have no chest pain or back pain. You now experience shortness of breath when walking up stairs. You do not feel more short of breath lying down and you do not wake suddenly from sleep gasping for breath. You have not noticed any swelling of your ankles nor any painful swelling of your calves.

You have lost your appetite and have lost a lot of weight but you are not sure how much. You have not had fevers or night sweats. You have high blood pressure. You have never been diagnosed with asthma, COPD, tuberculosis or HIV. You have never had a heart attack or a clot in your leg or lung. You take Losartan. You have no drug allergies. You have no family history of cancer.

You are now retired but worked for many years as a missionary in areas with a high prevalence of tuberculosis including India and Somalia. You may have been in contact with people with active tuberculosis but did not suffer any symptoms yourself. You had the recommended vaccinations prior to travel. You have never been exposed to asbestos. You smoked 10 cigarettes a day from your mid-teens until five years ago. You do not drink alcohol. You live with your wife of many years. Your wife has not been coughing.
If asked about your ideas, concerns and expectations please offer the information below

You think this might be cancer. Your wife is in the early stages of dementia and you are her main carer. You have no children and few local friends due to your itinerant lifestyle. You are concerned about who will look after your wife if this is something serious. You are expecting blood tests and scans but think this will take a long time on the NHS.

Mark Scheme: Chronic Cough

Task:	Achieved	Not Achieved
Introduces himself / herself		
Confirms patient details and purpose of consultation		
Established the main presenting complaint		
Explores symptom of cough - duration, whether cough is productive, coryzal symptoms		
Asks about red flags – weight loss, change in appetite, haemoptysis, night sweats		
Identify any exacerbating factors (e.g. dust, pets)		
Asks about associated features- chest pain and shortness of breath		
Exclude symptoms of heart failure, pulmonary embolism, infection		
Asks about past medical history specifically respiratory, cardiovascular problems, infections or causes of immunosuppression.		
Asks specifically about exposure to tuberculosis		
Asks about medications and allergies		
Asks about family history of lung cancer		
Asks about social history including alcohol and smoking		
Plans to examine or asks for examination findings		
Summarises findings concisely		
Able to provide appropriate differential diagnoses Lung cancer Tuberculosis		

Suggests appropriate investigations Routine blood tests - FBC - to check anaemia or other infection or immunosuppression, Blood film, CXR Sputum Culture Mantoux		
Appropriate management plan & follow-up 2 week referral pathway as per NICE guidelines May require support at home, can refer to community services for carers for wife.		
Acknowledges & addresses patient's ideas, concerns and expectations		
Gives patient opportunity to ask questions		
Examiner's Global Mark	/5	
Actor / Helper's Global Mark	/5	
Total Station Mark	/30	

Learning Points

- Lung cancer has a number of different presentations, it does not only occur in patients who have an extensive smoking history. In addition there are local and paraneoplastic complications associated with lung cancer, and complications related to metastases.

- It is essential to know and make a point of excluding red flag symptoms for lung cancer but try to avoid fixation error (focusing on one differential to the extent of being blind to alternative diagnoses). Think systematically and consider what other pathologies could cause the presenting symptoms.

- It is advisable to start with open questions, to allow the patient to tell you the story in their own words, but do push them to be specific on important points in your closed questioning.

Chapter 3: Neurology and Geriatrics

Case 1: Headache

Candidate's Instructions

You are the foundation year doctor working in General Practice and have been asked to see a 33 year old woman, Bekah who attends your GP practice with a headache.

After 6 minutes the examiner will stop you and ask you to summarise back your findings, suggest your differential diagnoses and your initial management plan.

Examiner's Instructions

A 33 year old woman, Bekah attends the GP practice with a headache. The candidate, is acting as the foundation year doctor, and has been asked to take a history from the patient.

After 6 minutes please stop the candidate at whatever stage they are and ask them to present the case with their primary differential diagnoses. Following this ask them what their next steps regarding investigations and management will be.

If they ask, give them the examination findings below:
Examination findings:
Louisa is comfortable at rest. Her observations are all in normal range, including her blood pressure.
She has no significant neurological signs on a full upper and lower limb and cranial nerve examination. All other systemic examinations are normal.
Questions to ask if there is time:
What are the diagnostic criteria for a migraine?

Actor's Instructions:

You are a 33 year old woman, Bekah and you have come to the GP because you have been having headaches for 3 months.
ONLY OFFER INFORMATION IF SPECIFICALLY ASKED

They are usually only on the left side of your head and are throbbing in nature. They are 8/10 in severity at worst. You have about 2-4 headaches per week and they last 2-3 hours. You can generally tell when you are about to have a headache as you have a strange visual sensation about 15 minutes beforehand. You have vomited a few times when you have had a headache and generally feel nauseous.

You think the headaches may be triggered by coffee or alcohol. Nothing particularly makes them worse but the pain does improve when lying down in a dark room. You take paracetamol every four hours during a headache. This helped initially but no longer has any effect.

You also have asthma which is generally well controlled with a blue inhaler if you get wheezy. You are also on the oral contraceptive pill for contraception.

Your mother suffers from tension headaches and you wonder if these are the same thing.

You work as a lawyer and live with your partner and your daughter. You have a very stressful case at the moment and are getting very little sleep.

If asked about your ideas, concerns and expectations please offer the information below

You are very worried as you have started to miss work because of your headaches and this is becoming very stressful. You would like some stronger pain relief and an explanation of what these headaches are and how they can be avoided.

Mark Scheme: Headache

Task:	Achieved	Not Achieved
Introduces himself / herself		
Confirms patient details and purpose of consultation		
Established the main presenting complaint		
Asks about site, radiation of headache and character and severity of the pain.		
Asks about timing of the headache. How quick is the onset? How long does it last for? How frequently do they have them?		
Asks if there has been any recent trauma, nausea or vomiting.		
Asks about aura or any preceding symptoms.		
Asks if they have any visual symptoms including photophobia and whether they have had a recent eye test.		
Asks about red flag symptoms including fever, neck stiffness, rash, seizures, limb weakness, weight loss		
Asks about triggers or anything that makes the headache worse or if anything improves the headache including lying in a dark room or analgesia		
Asks about medication and allergies, enquiring specifically about what analgesia they have been taking including dose and frequency.		
Asks about past medical history and family history		
Asks about social history, enquiring specifically about work, stress, alcohol, smoking and recreational drug use.		

Plans to examine or asks for examination findings		
Summarises findings concisely		
Able to provide appropriate differential diagnoses Migraine with aura Tension headaches Cluster headaches Drug related headaches (caffeine or analgesia) Raised intracranial pressure secondary to space occupying lesion. Exclude acute causes: Meningitis, Vascular (Subarachnoid haemorrhage)		
Suggests appropriate investigations Routine Bloods: FBC- identify markers of infection Imaging: CT scan		
Appropriate management plan & follow-up Avoid triggers Analgesia -working along the WHO Pain Ladder If migraine consider triptans or propanolol. Has considered that patient may have to use a different form of contraception to the oral contraceptive pill.		
Acknowledges & addresses patient's ideas, concerns and expectations		
Gives patient opportunity to ask questions		
Examiner's Global Mark	/5	
Actor / Helper's Global Mark	/5	
Total Station Mark	/30	

Learning Points

- Always consider red flag symptoms in any pain presentation. Are there any features that make this an acute emergency or make you suspect a malignancy?

- Don't be afraid to ask if anyone feels stressed or under pressure at home or work. You do not need to go into details or solve all their problems but it helps to get an idea of the bigger picture and may help explain their symptoms or behaviour. Make sure to do it sensitively and react compassionately.

- In any pain presentation make sure to take a thorough history of exactly which analgesia a patient has taken, at which dose and how frequently. This can give you an idea of the severity of the pain, if they are taking appropriate pain relief, whether they are taking therapeutic levels of a drug and also spot staggered overdoses.

Case 2: Stroke Management

Candidate's Instructions:

You are the foundation year doctor working in General Practice and have been asked to see a 75 year old lady, Mandy who has made an appointment with her GP as advised by her stroke consultant. She was discharged a week ago from the high intensity stroke unit where she spent two weeks following an acute ischaemic stroke. She had been told that her GP would arrange any further community follow up required.

Please take a history and address the patient's ideas, concerns and expectations. After 6 minutes the examiner will stop you and ask you to summarise back your findings, suggest your differential diagnoses and your initial management plan.

Examiner's Instructions:

A 75 year old lady Mandy has made an appointment as advised by her stroke consultant. She was discharged a week ago from the high intensity stroke unit where she spent two weeks following an acute ischaemic stroke. She had been told that her GP would arrange any further community follow up required.

The candidate, is acting as the foundation year doctor, and has been asked to take a brief history from the patient.

After 6 minutes please stop the candidate and ask them to present the case and propose their next steps regarding multidisciplinary management.

Questions to ask if there is time:
What is the classification system for stroke?

Actor's Instructions:

You are Mandy a 75 year old lady, who was discharged a week ago from the high intensity stroke unit where you spent two weeks following an ischaemic stroke. Your stroke consultant has advised you make an appointment with your GP to arrange community follow up.

ONLY OFFER INFORMATION IF SPECIFICALLY ASKED

You called an ambulance 2 weeks ago as you were not able to move your right leg and arm very well. Your family were also concerned about your speech, as it was slurred. Your were unable to tell what had happened. You had been well the previous day. You did not have a head injury or any loss of consciousness. They did a CT scan and they found you had a stroke, and you stayed for two weeks.

You have atrial fibrillation, high blood pressure and diabetes, but it is well controlled currently with medications. You don't remember your medications but the GP surgery have a record on the computer of your medicines. You don't have any drug allergies.

You are an ex-smoker, but stopped when you were 40yrs old, you used to smoke 20 per day for 20 years. You drink an occasional glass of wine. Your dad was diabetic and had lots of heart problems, he died aged 59 of a heart attack, you think.

The candidate will now have a discussion with the examiner. Following this they will take some time to address your ideas, concerns and expectations. You have some specific questions:

1. The last month has been a complete whirlwind and although you were given lots of information whilst in hospital, it has been difficult to take it all in. You feel there have been many technical terms used and everyone has

said the word stroke without fully explaining what it means. What is a stroke and why do I have to take aspirin?

2.   The stroke consultant mentioned that you would be able to tell me about community follow up and what can be offered? You feel like you could do with help with getting around and although you can walk, you feel very unsteady and have difficulty with the stairs and getting in and out of the bath.

3.   You were advised a soft diet when leaving hospital but you are getting fed up with pureed food and think your swallow is much better. Can you try solid food?

4.   Are you allowed to drive following your stroke? This is very important to you as you live in a small village and feel very isolated. You aren't able to go to your bridge group or any social gatherings and you feel very lonely. Your friends have visited a lot and done the shopping for you but you feel they don't understand what you are going through.

Mark Scheme: Stroke Management

Task:	Achieved	Not Achieved
Introduces himself / herself		
Confirms patient details and purpose of consultation		
Takes a brief history about their recent inpatient admission		
Asks about past medical history- asking specifically about hypertension, diabetes, high cholesterol, irregular heart rate, previous strokes.		
Asks about medications and allergies		
Asks about family history & social history including alcohol and smoking		
Summarises findings concisely		
Acknowledges & addresses patient's ideas, concerns and expectations		
Explains without using jargon what an ischaemic stroke is.		
Briefly explains the symptoms of a stroke.		
Explains to the patient how aspirin works to prevent further strokes.		
Recognises that the patient could benefit from physiotherapy and explains what a physiotherapist does.		
Explains that an occupational therapist may visit their home to assess what adjustments or equipment may be required.		

Informs the patient that it is possible to provide equipment/adjust homes to help with independent living - walking aids, handrailings		
Explains it is important to follow the soft diet until and assessment by a speech and language therapist who will assess what they can safely swallow. You will be able to arrange this.		
Informs the patient they are not allowed to drive for at least one month following a stroke. They may then be cleared by their doctor or be required to take a driving assessment.		
Explains to the patient it is their duty to tell the DVLA about any changes in their medical status including a stroke.		
Addresses patients loneliness: mentions a support service such as the stroke association who can provide individual advice and further information.		
Offers and information leaflet and suggests a review appointment to see how they are managing.		
Gives patient opportunity to ask questions		
Examiner's Global Mark	/5	
Actor / Helper's Global Mark	/5	
Total Station Mark	/30	

Learning Points

- Be careful not to use any jargon when explaining the roles of different professionals to patients. Whilst it is clear to us that an multidisciplinary team of an Occupational therapist, Physiotherapist and Speech and Language Therapist will be very useful to a patient it can leave them feeling very confused. Be sure to break down each team member's role and what help they can provide for their specific needs.

- A life changing diagnosis or condition can be terrifying and leave a patient feeling very isolated. Organisations such as the Stroke Association can help patients understand they are not alone and can provide valuable support as well as further resources and information sheets.

- When providing a lot of information in a single consultation it can be useful to offer them a further appointment in a few weeks to check in and see how they are getting along.

Case 3: Multiple Sclerosis

Candidate's Instructions

You are the foundation year doctor working in General Practice and have been asked to see a 38 year old lady Philippa who has presented to the GP surgery complaining of feeling unwell. You note from recent letters that she has recently been diagnosed with multiple sclerosis following two admissions to hospital under the Neurology team but has not seen her GP since her diagnosis.

Please take a history and address the patient's ideas, concerns and expectations. After 6 minutes the examiner will stop you and ask you to summarise back your findings, suggest your differential diagnoses and your initial management plan.

Examiner's Instructions

A 38 year old lady Philippa, has presented to the GP surgery complaining of feeling unwell. It is noted from recent letters that she has recently been diagnosed with multiple sclerosis following two admissions to hospital under the Neurology team but has not seen her GP since her diagnosis.

The candidate is an foundation year doctor in a GP practice and have been asked to carry out a consultation with Philippa, discuss her symptoms and address any concerns she may have.

After 6 minutes please stop the candidate and ask them to summarise the consultation and assessing patients understanding.

If they ask, give them the examination findings below:
Examination findings:
Philippa is comfortable at rest, observations are normal. Chest is clear with good air entry bilaterally. Throat is red with swollen tonsils, no pus. All other systemic examinations are normal.
Questions to ask if there is time:
What is the classification of Multiple Sclerosis?
What medications can be used acutely and to prevent relapses?

Actor's Instructions

You are Philippa, a 38 year old who has recently been diagnosed with Multiple sclerosis following two admissions to hospital. These admissions were prompted by an episode during which you experienced visual symptoms and an episode of right sided weakness, that has improved but remains, causing a slight limp.

ONLY OFFER INFORMATION IF SPECIFICALLY ASKED

You have come to the GP today because you have had a cough, runny nose and sore throat. You never really get unwell and you are worried this is related to your MS. You have not had a fever, your cough is non productive. You have not had any shortness of breath or chest pain. You have been taking lemsip which is helping.

You have no other medical problems and no drug allergies. There is no family history of multiple sclerosis. You are a teacher and have been in contact with lots of 6-7year olds who have come down with the flu. You do not smoke or drink. You live with your fiance.

You have not felt fatigued or in pain recently. You are not experiencing any tingling or pins and needles. Your eye symptoms have resolved. You have no incontinence or urinary symptoms.

If asked about your ideas, concerns and expectations please offer the information below

When asked by your GP what you know about MS, confess that you are feeling quite overwhelmed by all the information you have been given and feeling quite confused. You are not sure about which symptoms could be due to MS.

1. When the GP/candidate explains that this is unlikely related to your MS, ask which things you should look out

for and what to do if you get these symptoms. Can the GP provide new medications?

2. You wonder if your leg is going to get any better at all as the limp is causing quite an inconvenience. Will all new symptoms continue to get worse?

3. Another big concern you have is your job. You are a teacher in a busy primary school and have to move classrooms to teach different classes, which is difficult with your leg. Will you have to quit your job?

4. Since your diagnosis you have been feeling very anxious and worried. You are struggling to sleep at night because you worry about the future- you don't want to have to use a wheelchair or have carers.

Mark Scheme: Multiple Sclerosis

Task:	Achieved	Not Achieved
Introduces himself / herself		
Confirms patient details and purpose of consultation		
Established the main presenting complaint		
Elicits her symptoms		
Asks about past medical history		
Asks about medications and allergies		
Asks about family history & social history including alcohol and smoking		
Plans to examine or asks for examination findings		
Explains that her symptoms sound like an upper respiratory tract infection and are unlikely to be related to her multiple sclerosis		
Acknowledges & addresses patient's ideas, concerns and expectations		
Briefly gives an explanation of what multiple sclerosis is.		
Asks the patient what symptoms she has experienced and explains what other symptoms to look out for- eye symptoms, motor/sensory problems, incontinence		
Explains to the patient that she should contact either her GP or MS nurse if she has any further symptoms. However, it tends to be your neurologist who decided on medications.		
Explained that although some symptoms of MS resolve completely some can remain.		
Explains to the patient that it should be possible to make arrangements at work help her (for example- teaching all her classes in the same classroom). Suggest making an appointment with headteacher or if possible disability officer to talk about her MS and to see what arrangements are possible.		
Addresses patient's social support: mentions a support service such as the multiple sclerosis trust who can provide individual support and further information.		
Appropriate management plan & follow-up		

Offers a review appointment to see how they are managing. Review of her sleep and symptoms of depression at the next consultation		
Summarises the consultation to the patient concisely		
Assesses patient's understanding of the information given to her		
Gives patient opportunity to ask questions		
Examiner's Global Mark	/5	
Actor / Helper's Global Mark	/5	
Total Station Mark	/30	

Learning Points

- If you are asked to discuss a patient's condition or new diagnosis, it is essential to start is by establishing what they know so far and what they would like to know. This can help provide a structure for you explanation and help fill the gaps in their knowledge.

- A new diagnosis of a progressive or chronic condition can be terrifying. Showing empathy and kindness are key. You won't be able to answer all their questions about the future in a short consultation but reassuring them of the support they have and making them aware of the team available will help address their fears.

- When providing a lot of information in a single consultation it can be useful to offer them a further appointment in a few weeks to check in and see how they are getting along. Also remember patients with chronic conditions are at a higher risk of developing depression so it is good to review their mood regularly.

Case 4: Memory Loss

Candidate's Instructions

You are the foundation year doctor working in General Practice and have been asked to Colleen who has presented to the GP surgery as she is worried about her husband's progressing confusion. Please take a collateral history from the relative.

After 6 minutes the examiner will stop you and ask you to summarise back your findings, suggest your differential diagnoses and your initial management plan.

Examiner's Instructions

Colleen has presented to the GP surgery as she is worried about her husband's progressing confusion.

The candidate, is acting as the foundation year doctor, and has been asked to take a history from the patient's wife.

After 6 minutes please stop the candidate at whatever stage they are and ask them to present the case with their primary differential diagnoses. Following this ask them what their next steps regarding investigations and management will be.
Questions to ask if there is time:
What will a referral to memory clinic provide for this patient?

Actor's Instructions

You are Colleen and have presented to the GP surgery, as you are worried about his progressing confusion. He is now 82 years old. *ONLY OFFER INFORMATION IF SPECIFICALLY ASKED*

You are worried about your husband as he growing increasingly confused. You have come in today as he was recently aggressive towards you and you feel you cannot cope anymore. This has been going on for many years. You first noticed your husband's memory was awry 4 years ago when he began forgetting simple things like where he had put his keys. This has got worse and now he is beginning to forget friends and family.

He is often awake at night and often calls out during his sleep. He gets agitated very easily. He does not seem depressed or flat in his mood. His cognition does not seem to fluctuate through the day. He has no hallucinations.

This seems to be have been a slow progressive worsening rather than a sudden deterioration. There have been no recent signs of infection - no cough, no fevers, no urinary incontinence, no diarrhoea.

His mobility is fine and he is able to take himself to the toilet but there have been accidents recently. However you are his main carer and have to help him with washing and dressing. You prepare his food now, as there have been dangerous occurrences where he has left the gas on and recently you found him wandering outside alone with no good reason. This has changed your life as he no longer cooks for himself and this was a huge passion of his.

He has a past medical history of high blood pressure for which he is on Amlodipine. He has no drug allergies.

He is a retired lawyer and did not smoke or drink very much. You do not have any family around, as they have moved to Australia, and friends have their own problems that have come with age.

If asked about your ideas, concerns and expectations please offer the information below

You are worried about your husband's health and safety, as you can not leave him in the house alone anymore. You fear it may be dementia. In addition it has impacted your life greatly and at your age are finding it difficult to cope at home, especially with controlling his behaviour and aggression, but also just with washing and dressing him.

Mark Scheme: Memory Loss

Task:	Achieved	Not Achieved
Introduces himself / herself		
Confirms patient details and purpose of consultation		
Established the main presenting complaint and chronicity		
Elicits sleep disturbances and behavioural disturbances		
Establishes lack of hallucinations		
Establishes lack of fluctuance throughout day.		
Establishes lack of stepwise decline		
Establishes lack of recent trigger (infection)		
Discusses impact on ADL's (cleaning, washing, toileting)		
Establishes dangerous symptoms and safety issues (regarding gas cooker and wandering)		
Asks about past medical history		
Asks about medications and allergies		
Asks about family history & social history including prior occupation, alcohol and smoking.		
Asks about support from family and friends		
Summarises findings concisely		
Able to provide appropriate differential diagnoses Alzheimer's Disease Vascular Dementia Lewy Body Dementia		
Suggests appropriate investigations Routine bloods: FBC: review inflammatory markers, B12/folate, Thyroid function, Renal function. Urine dip Blood sugar Imaging: CT head		
Appropriate management plan & follow-up Offers a review appointment to see how they are managing and also to formally examine Mr Collier Referral to memory clinic Referral to community services for potential carers to help at home e.g. physiotherapy and occupational health		

Acknowledges & addresses patient's ideas, concerns and expectations		
Gives patient opportunity to ask questions		
Examiner's Global Mark	/5	
Actor / Helper's Global Mark	/5	
Total Station Mark	/30	

Learning Points

- There are subtle differences within dementia. A good way to separate Alzheimer's Disease, vascular dementia and Lewy-Body Dementia is to think about the temporal pattern of the disease (progressive, step-wise and fluctuating deterioration respectively).

- It is important to be aware of the effect dementia has on family members who are often the principal carers. With an aging population the role of families to deliver care has increased. There is now a need for clinicians to consider the wellbeing of the patient's relatives and the mental and physical effects of the illness on their own health.

- Within the community it is important to be aware of community geriatric and memory services and the role the MDT can play. The memory teams can consist of geriatricians, nurse specialists, psychaitrists and pyschologists.

Case 5: Multiple Falls & Medication Review

Candidate's Instructions

You are the foundation year doctor working in General Practice and have been asked to see a 78 year old man Kamran who has been sent in by his wife to the GP clinic after he suffered a fall this morning. Please take a history and perform medication review.

After 6 minutes the examiner will stop you and ask you to summarise back your findings, suggest your differential diagnoses and your initial management plan.

Examiner's instructions

A 78 year old man Kamran , has been sent in by his wife after she witnessed him fall this morning when he got out of bed. This is not the first time it has happened and she is starting to get worried.

The candidate, is acting as the foundation year doctor Doctor, and has been asked to take a history from the patient.

After 6 minutes please stop the candidate and ask them to perform a medication review. Following this ask them what their differential diagnoses are and their next steps regarding investigations and management will be.

If they ask, give them the examination findings below:
Examination findings:
Kamran is comfortable at rest, his lying blood pressure is 136/76 and his standing blood pressure is 104/62. All other observations are normal. All other systemic examinations are normal.

Questions to ask if there is time:
What is the definition of postural hypotension?
What are causes of postural hypotension?

Actor's instructions:

You are Kamran, a 78 year old who has been sent in by your wife as she is worried about the increase in falls he has had recently.

ONLY OFFER INFORMATION IF SPECIFICALLY ASKED

Your last fall was this morning as you were getting out of bed. You felt well going to bed last night and had a good sleep, but when you got out of bed, you felt dizzy and felt your legs give way as you collapsed onto the floor.

You did not lose consciousness and did not hit your head or have any other injuries except for a bruise on your left arm. It took you a minute to compose yourself but you were able to stand up and get about afterwards.

In the last 2 weeks, this is the fourth time this has happened. It is similar each time. You are normally in a sitting or lying position and when you stand up, you have dizziness and fall. You feel well otherwise.

You have not noticed any weakness, pins and needles, speech difficulties, visual disturbances, fevers, sweats, chest pains, shortness of breath or palpitations. There has been no change in your ability to walk smoothly. Your bowel motions and urinary habits have not changed either.

You are a retired teacher who lives with his wife in a bungalow. You lead an active lifestyle and play golf 3 times a week. You drink a glass of red wine every night after dinner. You are an ex smoker, you stopped at the age of 52 when you lost one of your close friends due to a lung disease.

Your father suffered from Parkinson's disease which started around the age of 75 for him.

Your medical history includes type 2 diabetes for which you take Metformin 1gram twice daily and high blood pressure for which you take Amlodipine 10mg once daily and Ramipril 5mg once daily. You are allergic to Penicillin and find Ibuprofen upsets your stomach. The GP increased the dose of Amlodipine from 5mg about 3 weeks ago.

If asked about your ideas, concerns and expectations please offer the information below
You are not very concerned as you feel it is a normal part of getting old, but your wife is very concerned and would not have been happy if you did not come today. You are hoping the doctor will say everything is fine and you can go home and reassure her.

Mark Scheme: Multiple Falls

Task:	Achieved	Not Achieved
Introduces himself / herself		
Confirms patient details and purpose of consultation		
Established the main presenting complaint		
Assesses pre, during and post-fall events		
Asks about symptoms of chest pain, palpitations, shortness of breath, sweating		
Asks about symptoms of headache, visual disturbances, focal weakness, slurred speech, urinary incontinence, seizure activity, gait disturbance		
Asks about head injury and loss of consciousness (mechanism, duration, witness)		
Assesses any previous falls and their nature (whether similar or different)		
Asks about red flag symptoms: fevers, weight loss, night sweats, loss of appetite		
Asks about infective symptoms: cough, dysuria, frequency, vomiting, diarrhoea		
Asks about past medical history specifically previous stroke, ischaemic heart disease, hypertension, Parkinson's disease		
Asks about medications and allergies specifically asking about recent changes made to medications		
Asks about family history & social history including alcohol and smoking		
Plans to examine or asks for examination findings		
Summarises findings concisely		
Able to provide appropriate differential diagnoses Postural Hypotension Cardiac Arrhythmia Parkinson's Disease		
Suggests appropriate investigations Lying and standing blood pressure Blood sugar ECG 24 hour ECG and blood pressure monitoring		
Appropriate management plan & follow-up		

Suggests reducing dose/withholding anti-hypertensives Offers a review appointment to see how they are managing.		
Acknowledges & addresses patient's ideas, concerns and expectations Gives patient opportunity to ask questions		
Examiner's Global Mark	/5	
Actor / Helper's Global Mark	/5	
Total Station Mark	/30	

Learning points

- In the elderly patient with falls, postural (Orthostatic) hypotension often due to anti-hypertensives is an important and common diagnosis to rule out. Polypharmacy in general is an issue and can lead to worsening falls. Careful review of medications, their timings and their combined interactions should be performed regularly on the wards.

- Parkinson's disease and many of the drug treatments for it may also cause postural hypotension. Close questioning of the features of tremor, rigidity and bradykinesia should be sought out.

- Consider referral to hospital specialties such as Cardiology, Geriatrics and Neurology for ruling out relevant differentials such as paroxysmal arrhythmias and Parkinson's disease.

Chapter 4: Gastroenterology & Colorectal Surgery

Case 1: Change in Bowel Habit

Candidate's Instructions

You are the foundation year doctor working in General Practice and have been asked to see a 68-year-old man, Rafael who has presented to the GP surgery complaining of change in his bowel habit. Please take a full history.

After 6 minutes the examiner will stop you and ask you to summarise back your findings, suggest your differential diagnoses and your initial management plan.

Examiner's Instructions

A 68-year-old man Rafael has presented to the GP surgery complaining of change in his bowel habit.

The candidate, is acting as the foundation year doctor, and has been asked to take a history from the patient.

After 6 minutes please stop the candidate and ask them to present the case with their primary differential diagnoses. Following this ask them what their next steps regarding investigations and management will be.
If they ask, give them the examination findings below:
Examination findings:
Mr Smith looks thin and pale on examination, but comfortable. His observations are normal. His abdomen is soft, no obvious masses are felt. Digital rectal examination is normal.
All other systemic examinations are normal.
Questions to ask if there is time:
What is the staging system for colorectal cancer?
How can you manage a patient with colorectal cancer?

Actor's Instructions:

You are a 68-year-old man Rafael, who has come to the GP surgery complaining of diarrhoea for 3 months.

ONLY OFFER INFORMATION IF SPECIFICALLY ASKED

You now regularly pass very loose stools, but on occasion it has been watery. You open your bowels 1-2 times per day, and you feel like you are completely emptying your bowels. In the past 2 weeks there has been a handful of occasions where you have noticed some fresh blood mixed in your stool. There is no mucus in your stool and you have not had abdominal pain. You previously had quite regular in bowel movements and rarely had diarrhoea.

You have been feeling more tired than normal, but you think this is because you are renovating your house. You have had to buy smaller clothes recently and realized you have had to tighten your belt 2 notches, but again you think this is because you have been busy renovating your house.

You have not made any dietary changes and have not been travelling in the past year.

You consider yourself a healthy person and are unaware of any physical health problems. You are not on any regular medications. You have never suffered from anything similar in the past.

You drink alcohol occasionally (approximately 3-4 pints per week) and smoke 5/day for the past 30 years. Your parents are both deceased – your mum died of a stroke when she was 80, and your father died of a 'blood clot on the lung' when he was 60.

If asked about your ideas, concerns and expectations please offer the information below

You say now that your father had bowel cancer as well when he died. When you remember this, you begin to get quite anxious and tearful. You admit to the doctor that you are worried about cancer and did not know what to do.

Mark Scheme - Change in Bowel Habit

Task:	Achieved	Not Achieved
Introduces himself / herself		
Confirms patient details and purpose of consultation		
Established the main presenting complaint		
Elicits circumstances of change in bowel habit		
Asks about their normal bowel movements		
Asks about tenesmus		
Asks about abdominal pain		
Asks about rectal bleeding - colour and if mixed in stool or in pan or on tissue.		
Asks about red flag symptoms - weight loss, loss of appetite, lethargy, night sweats, fevers		
Asks about other causes of change in bowel habit (i.e. recent travel, change in diet)		
Asks about past medical history		
Asks about medications and allergies		
Asks about family history of cancer & social history including alcohol and smoking		
Plans to examine or asks for examination findings		
Summarises findings concisely		
Able to provide appropriate differential diagnoses Bowel cancer Inflammatory Bowel disease		

Infection - campylobacter, shigella		
Suggests appropriate investigations Routine bloods - FBC - anaemia, Renal function, Liver function, Faecal occult blood, Carcinoembryonic antigen (tumour marker) Stool culture Imaging: Endoscopy/Colonoscopy and CT scan		
Appropriate management plan & follow-up Urgent 2 week wait referral to gastrointestinal surgeons Offers a review appointment to see how they are managing.		
Acknowledges & addresses patient's ideas, concerns and expectations		
Gives patient opportunity to ask questions		
Examiner's Global Mark	/5	
Actor / Helper's Global Mark	/5	
Total Station Mark	/30	

Learning Points

- Knowledge of the two-week-wait suspected cancer referral pathway is essential here and when it is appropriate.

  - >40 with unexplained weight loss and abdominal pain
  - >50 with unexplained rectal bleeding
  - >60 with iron-deficiency anaemia, **or** changes in bowel habit, **or** tests show occult blood in faeces

- It can be difficult to reassure a patient when they are worried about cancer and you as the doctor, are referring them for suspected cancer investigations. However, it is important to be open with patients and explain to them why you are referring them.

- When asking about family history it is important to remember that the patient may not always realize what is significant, so to ask directly if there is a history of cancer.

Case 2: Inflammatory Bowel Disease

Candidate's Instructions

You are the foundation year doctor working in General Practice and have been asked to see a 20 year old man Dawson who has presented to the GP surgery complaining of abdominal pain. Please take a full history.

After 6 minutes the examiner will stop you and ask you to summarise back your findings, suggest your differential diagnoses and your initial management plan.

Examiner's Instructions

A 20 year old man Dawson has presented to the GP surgery complaining of abdominal pain.

The candidate, is acting as the foundation year doctor, and has been asked to take a history from the patient.

After 6 minutes please stop the candidate and ask them to present the case with their primary differential diagnoses. Following this ask them what their next steps regarding investigations and management will be.

If they ask, give them the examination findings below:
Examination findings:
Dawson is comfortable at rest, his observations are normal. His abdomen is soft and non tender currently, with no organomegaly or masses felt. All other systemic examinations are normal.
Questions to ask if there is time:
What are the main differences between Crohn's disease and Ulcerative Colitis?

Actor's Instructions

You are a 20-year-old man Dawson, who has come to see your GP as you have had abdominal pain for the past 3 years.

ONLY OFFER INFORMATION IF SPECIFICALLY ASKED

You experience it 3-4 times per week. You feel it start on the left lower side of your abdomen, but it radiates to the right side. It is a cramp-like pain that comes in waves, most severe is an 8/10. It usually comes on in the afternoon and lasts a few hours, and has started to affect your studies as you often have to leave college early. You have tried taking painkillers, like paracetamol, and avoiding certain foods but nothing seems to work. With the pain you also experience diarrhoea about 2-3 times a day. Your stools are very loose, and has small amounts of fresh blood or mucus in it. You deny faecal urgency but you do sometimes have the urge to pass stool, even after you have gone.

You very occasionally have mouth ulcers. You deny any joint problems or skin rashes. You feel very lethargic. You deny any recent travel.

You have no past medical history and take no regular medications and you have no drug allergies.

You drink alcohol occasionally and are a non-smoker. You are a student at college. Your mother and older sister both have ulcerative colitis.

If asked about your ideas, concerns and expectations please offer the information below

You are very worried that this could be ulcerative colitis as your mother and sister were also in their early 20s when they were diagnosed. You are anxious as you have seen how the disease affects them and the different medications they have to take. You are wanting to have investigations be carried out and be referred to a gastroenterologist today. You feel a follow up appointment with the GP is pointless and your next appointment should be with the specialist.

Mark Scheme: Inflammatory Bowel Disease

Task:	Achieved	Not Achieved
Introduces himself / herself		
Confirms patient details and purpose of consultation		
Established the main presenting complaint		
Takes thorough history about abdominal pain - ascertains site of pain and radiation, timing, onset and character of pain.		
Asks about diarrhoea		
Asks about blood or mucus in stool		
Asks about faecal urgency or tenesmus		
Asks about red flag symptoms - weight loss, loss of appetite, lethargy, night sweats, fevers		
Asks about extraintestinal features, such as joint or skin problems		
Asks about past medical history, specifically other autoimmune diseases		
Asks about medications and allergies		
Asks about family history, including IBD, coeliac or colorectal cancer & social history including alcohol and smoking		
Asks about how their symptoms affects their daily life		
Plans to examine or asks for examination findings		
Summarises findings concisely		
Able to provide appropriate differential diagnoses Inflammatory Bowel disease Irritable bowel syndrome Coeliac disease		
Suggests appropriate investigations Routine bloods- FBC - anaemia, inflammatory markers including ESR, CRP. Specific tests - faecal calprotectin Stool Culture Imaging- Endoscopy/Colonoscopy		
Appropriate management plan & follow-up Offers a follow up appointment to discuss results and possibility of further referral to gastroenterology		

Acknowledges & addresses patient's ideas, concerns and expectations		
Gives patient opportunity to ask questions		
Examiner's Global Mark	/5	
Actor / Helper's Global Mark	/5	
Total Station Mark	/30	

Learning Points

- It is important to be aware of symptoms that would require you to arrange emergency admission to hospital, even if there is no established diagnosis:
  More than 6 stools a day plus one of the following:
  - Pyrexia
  - Tachycardia
  - Anaemia (Hb<10.5g/100mL)
  - Erythrocyte sedimentation rate >30mm/hour
  - Blood in the stool

- If unsure about a diagnosis, you can always ask the patient what their ideas, concerns and expectations are, as they may reveal more information that will help guide your differential diagnosis.

- Patients may be focussed on a specific diagnosis and can assume they will be referred immediately to a specialist. It is important to explain that initial investigations can be done in primary care to get a better idea of what is going on before referring onto secondary care.

Case 3: Alcoholic Liver Disease

Candidate's Instructions

You are the foundation year doctor working in General Practice and have been asked to see a 45 year old gentleman Harry who has presented to the GP surgery as he would like to cut down on his alcohol intake. Please take a full history.

After 6 minutes the examiner will stop you and ask you to summarise back your findings, suggest your differential diagnoses and your initial management plan.

Examiner's Instructions

A 45 year old gentleman Harry has presented to the GP surgery as he would like to cut down on his alcohol intake.

The candidate, is acting as the foundation year doctor and has been asked to take a history from the patient.

After 6 minutes please stop the candidate and ask them to present the case with their primary differential diagnoses. Following this ask them what their next steps regarding investigations and management will be.

If they ask, give them the examination findings below:
Examination findings:

Harry is comfortable at rest and is not confused, with normal observations. There are no peripheral signs of chronic liver disease including dupytrens contractures or spider naevi. His abdomen is soft and there is no tenderness and no evidence of hepatomegaly or jaundice. No evidence of peripheral neuropathy.
All other systemic examinations are normal.
Questions to ask if there is time:
What is Wernicke's encephalopathy and Korsakoffs?
What are the signs of alcohol withdrawal?

Actor's Instructions

You are a 45 year old gentleman Harry who has presented to the GP surgery as he would like to cut down on his alcohol intake.

ONLY OFFER INFORMATION IF SPECIFICALLY ASKED

You feel quite nervous about coming in to see the GP and are embarrassed that things have gotten this bad. Your girlfriend has recently given you an ultimatum that you must either seek help or she will leave.

You have always enjoyed a drink since you were younger and you feel 'you have always been a good laugh', but you have never had an alcohol problem in the past. You started drinking more about a year ago when you had a difficult time at work, following being suspended.

It used to start with having a glass of wine when you came home from work, and escalated to drinking a bottle of wine every day. However, in the past 3 months you have had to take many sick days as you felt too unwell to go in, and your boss has had several conversations with you about this, the most recent being last week where he told you that he has smelled alcohol on you and he was concerned so he has told you to take time off as leave.

You have found yourself having to have a drink in the morning to help you start your day. Usually this is a can of cider. You do not drink that much spirits. If asked to quantify exactly how much you drink you have 1 bottle of wine a day, and go through a 8-pack of cider in a week.

You deny any other drug use, but you smoke 20/day. You deny any other physical health problems or history of mental health. You have not had any problems with legal authorities.

You have no symptoms of gastritis, memory loss/confusion, no pins and needles in your hands and feet, and you do not experience palpitations.

If asked about your ideas, concerns and expectations please offer the information below
Your relationship with your girlfriend has become very difficult and you find you now mostly argue about your drinking, as she wants you to stop. She is upset as she is worried that you will lose your job and she will not be able to support you both. You feel very guilty and ashamed that she feels this way, but you get annoyed because that is all she says to you now.

You are willing to seek help as you have realised you need to change.

Mark Scheme: Alcoholic Liver disease

Task:	Achieved	Not Achieved
Introduces himself / herself		
Confirms patient details and purpose of consultation		
Established the main presenting complaint		
Finds out how long he has had a drinking problem		
Enquires about triggers for increasing alcohol use		
Asks about what/how much he drinks		
Uses the CAGE questionnaire, or another tool to assess if there is an alcohol problem Asks if they feel they should cut down on their drinking Asks if they have been annoyed by other people criticizing their drinking Asks if they feel guilty about their drinking Asks if they have had to drink first thing in the morning		
Asks if they have missed work or other responsibilities because of alcohol		
Asks if alcohol has put strain on personal relationships		
Enquires about other drugs & smoking		
Enquires about problems with legal authorities		
Asks about their motivation to stop drinking alcohol		
Asks about alcohol related symptoms: gastritis, peripheral sensory neuropathy, memory problems, palpitations.		
Asks about past medical history, medications and allergies, family history.		
Plans to examine or asks for examination findings		
Summarises findings concisely		
Appropriate management plan & follow-up States wants to make follow up appointment to discuss this further Signposts to written/online advice about alcohol misuse in the meantime		
Remains non-judgemental		

Acknowledges & addresses patient's ideas, concerns and expectations		
Gives patient opportunity to ask questions		
Examiner's Global Mark	/5	
Actor / Helper's Global Mark	/5	
Total Station Mark	/30	

Learning Points

- The CAGE questionnaire is a quick and easy tool to identify if a person has a significant alcohol problem. There are other tools, such as the AUDIT tool, however this takes several minutes to complete.

- Offering advice about alcohol misuse will require much more than a single appointment, so it is imperative to take a full history and make follow up appointments to further discuss.

- It is important to remain non-judgemental when discussing such sensitive topics. However, you must also establish a clear history and will need to ask sensitive questions.

Case 4: Gastritis

Candidate's Instructions

You are the foundation year doctor working in General Practice and have been asked to see a 24 year old gentleman William who has presented to the GP surgery complaining of abdominal pain. Please take a full history.

After 6 minutes the examiner will stop you and ask you to summarise back your findings, suggest your differential diagnoses and your initial management plan.

Examiner's Instructions

A 24 year old gentleman, Mr Williams, has presented to the GP surgery complaining of abdominal pain.

The candidate, is acting as the foundation year doctor and has been asked to take a history from the patient.

After 6 minutes please stop the candidate and ask them to present the case with their primary differential diagnoses. Following this ask them what their next steps regarding investigations and management will be.
If they ask, give them the examination findings below:
Examination findings:
All other systemic examinations are normal.
Questions to ask if there is time:
What is triple therapy for helicobacter pylori?

Actor's Instructions

You are a 24-year-old man William who has been experiencing intermittent abdominal pain for the past month.

ONLY OFFER INFORMATION IF SPECIFICALLY ASKED
You feel it across the upper part of your abdomen and it is most severe in the middle. Occasionally it radiates to lower abdomen. You describe it as a sharp burning pain. You rate the pain 5/10. It happens several times a week and it comes on gradually and lasts for 1-2 hours. It goes away with paracetamol or ibuprofen.

You feel nauseous with the pain but no vomiting and you have not brought up blood. No constipation/diarrhoea, no urinary symptoms, no chest pain, no shortness of breath, no lethargy, no weight loss.
You are fit and well with no other medical problems or regular medications. You have no drug allergies. You are a non-smoker. You usually drink about 5 pints a week, and when asked about alcohol you say you think the pain is worse after a night out.

If asked about diet you often get takeaways and you have noticed that the symptoms are worse after this, especially curry. You deny eating citrus foods.
If asked about your ideas, concerns and expectations please offer the information below
If asked what your concerns or expectations are, state that you are not sure what the problem is but you want to know if you need further tests or medication.

Mark Scheme: Gastritis

Task:	Achieved	Not Achieved
Introduces himself / herself		
Confirms patient details and purpose of consultation		
Established the main presenting complaint		
Ascertains site of pain and radiation		
Elicits timing, onset and character of pain		
Asks specifically about radiation through to back		
Asks about associated symptoms - nausea, vomiting, haematemesis, chest pain, shortness of breath.		
Asks about exacerbating features - weight, diet, alcohol		
Asks about red flag symptoms - weight loss, loss of appetite, lethargy, night sweats, fevers		
Asks about past medical history specifically NSAID use		
Asks about medications and allergies		
Asks about family history & social history including alcohol and smoking		
Plans to examine or asks for examination findings		
Summarises findings concisely		
Able to provide appropriate differential diagnoses Dyspepsia Peptic Ulcer disease Gastroesophageal Reflux Helicobacter Infection		

Suggests appropriate investigations Routine bloods - FBC - anaemia C13 breath test Imaging - Endoscopy - for biopsies		
Offers lifestyle advice Reduce or stop alcohol Advises dietary changes - avoid spicy, fatty & citrus		
Appropriate management plan & follow-up Suggests gavison for symptomatic relief Trial of a protein pump inhibitor e.g omeprazole Advises to return if no improvement in one month or sooner if symptoms worsen or become more frequent		
Acknowledges & addresses patient's ideas, concerns and expectations		
Gives patient opportunity to ask questions		
Examiner's Global Mark	/5	
Actor / Helper's Global Mark	/5	
Total Station Mark	/30	

Learning Points

- When a patient presents with gastritis, it is important to ask about any alarming features that would warrant further investigation, including haemoptysis, dysphagia or an upper abdominal mass. It is important to consider cardiac causes for the pain as indigestion can mimic angina.

- It is important to explore a patient's social history and identify if any particular lifestyle factors could be contributing to the patient's symptoms, and therefore aid with diagnosis and management. Before rushing to invasive investigations it is right to try and address and modifiable lifestyle factors.

- Remember to ask patients to return for a review if their symptoms do not improve. If there is no improvement after 1 month PPI, they will have to test for Helicobacter pylori.

Case 5: Rectal Bleeding

Candidate's Instructions

You are the foundation year doctor working in General Practice and have been asked to see a 37 year old gentleman Sam who has presented to the GP surgery complaining of rectal bleeding. Please take a full history.

After 6 minutes the examiner will stop you and ask you to summarise back your findings, suggest your differential diagnoses and your initial management plan.

Examiner's Instructions

A 37 year old gentleman Sam has presented to the GP surgery complaining of rectal bleeding.

The candidate, is acting as the foundation year doctor, and has been asked to take a history from the patient.

After 6 minutes please stop the candidate at whatever stage they are and ask them to present the case with their primary differential diagnoses. Following this ask them what their next steps regarding investigations and management will be.

If they ask, give them the examination findings below:

Examination findings:

Sam is comfortable at rest. Digital rectal examination is uncomfortable for the patient and there is no evidence of haemorrhoids. All other systemic examinations are normal.

Questions to ask if there is time:

What is the classification for the degree of haemorrhoids?
What is the surgical treatment of haemorrhoids?

Actor's Instructions

A 37 year old gentleman Sam, has presented to the GP surgery complaining of rectal bleeding.

ONLY OFFER INFORMATION IF SPECIFICALLY ASKED
This has been for the past month and happens intermittently. It is bright red blood and you notice it on wiping mostly, however recently you have noticed it in the toilet pan, which has made you more concerned. You do not think the blood is mixed in with stool. If asked about change in bowel habit, you cannot identify any obvious change. You have not had any diarrhoea. You have not been constipated but occasionally you do strain which is associated with pain followed by itching. You deny any black tarry stools, mucus in the stool, abdominal pain, or weight loss.
You report you eat a reasonably healthy diet. Only if asked directly, you do not eat enough fibre nor drink a lot of water.

You are a fit and healthy person. You have seasonal asthma and have inhalers blue and brown. You do not have any allergies. You are a non-smoker and drink very occasionally. You do a lot of exercise and work as a builder. You have no family history of bowel disease.

If asked about your ideas, concerns and expectations please offer the information below
You are worried about the bleeding and would like to know if it is something sinister and if there is anything you can do to manage it.

Mark Scheme: Rectal Bleeding

Task:	Achieved	Not Achieved
Introduces himself / herself		
Confirms patient details and purpose of consultation		
Established the main presenting complaint		
Asks about straining		
Asks about pain on passing stools		
Asks about anal itch		
Asks about abdominal pain		
Asks about red flag symptoms - weight loss, loss of appetite, lethargy, night sweats, fevers, change in bowel habit		
Asks patient about fibre & fluid intake		
Asks about past medical history		
Asks about medications and allergies		
Asks about family history & social history including alcohol and smoking		
Plans to examine or asks for examination findings		
Summarises findings concisely		
Able to provide appropriate differential diagnoses Haemorrhoids Anal Fissure Inflammatory Bowel disease		
Suggests appropriate investigations Bloods - exclude IBD		

Imaging - Rigid sigmoidoscopy		
Offers lifestyle advice Drinking plenty of water Eating lots of fibre rich foods Wiping hard makes haemorrhoids worse Warm baths can help		
Appropriate management plan & follow-up Explains need for soft stool to allow haemorrhoids to heal Offers topical creams/suppositories for symptom relief Offers a review appointment to see how they are managing.		
Acknowledges & addresses patient's ideas, concerns and expectations		
Gives patient opportunity to ask questions		
Examiner's Global Mark	/5	
Actor / Helper's Global Mark	/5	
Total Station Mark	/30	

Learning Points

- Remember to consider that many different factors can lead to haemorrhoids, not just constipation and straining when opening bowels, including age, raised intra-abdominal pressure (pregnancy, ascites, pelvic mass), chronic cough, heavy lifting, low fibre diet.

- Management of haemorrhoids is predominantly lifestyle advice, such as dietary advice, and it is important to emphasize to the patient that these changes will be long-term to reduce recurrence of haemorrhoids.

- It is important to ask about red flag symptoms for lower gastrointestinal cancers to ensure you do not miss something sinister, even if they fall outside the typical age group. Urgent referral via the 2 week wait cancer pathway is recommended for patients aged 40 and over who present with rectal bleeding with a change of bowel habit with looser stools and/or increased stool frequency that has been present for six weeks or more.

Chapter 5: Other Surgery

Case 1: Leg Pain

Candidate's Instructions

You are the foundation year doctor working in General Practice and have been asked to see A 67 year old gentleman Roland who has presented to the GP surgery complaining of a two week history of pain in his right leg. Please take a full history.

After 6 minutes the examiner will stop you and ask you to summarise back your findings, suggest your differential diagnoses and your initial management plan.

Examiner's Instructions

A 67 year old gentleman Roland, has presented to the GP surgery complaining of a two week history of pain in his right leg.

The candidate, is acting as the foundation year doctor, and has been asked to take a history from the patient.

After 6 minutes please stop the candidate at whatever stage they are and ask them to present the case with their primary differential diagnoses. Following this ask them what their next steps regarding investigations and management will be.

If they ask, give them the examination findings below:
Examination findings:
Roland is comfortable at rest, his BP 145/89, other observations are normal. He has normal pulses bilaterally from carotids to the dorsalis pedis. There are no ulcers noted and his legs are warm and well perfused with normal sensation. All other systemic examinations are normal.

Questions to ask if there is time:
What are the 6Ps of a critical ischaemic leg?
What is Buerger's angle?

Actor's Instructions:

You are a 67 year old gentleman Rowland who has presented to the GP surgery complaining of a two week history of pain in his right leg.

ONLY OFFER INFORMATION IF SPECIFICALLY ASKED
This pain has been getting progressively worse. You first noticed a cramping like pain in your right thigh when you were playing a round of golf with your former colleagues, and you found it difficult to walk up a hill on the green. You needed to take rest for a few moments on the second hole, some thirty metres or so. When you sat down to rest, the pain went away within a few minutes.

You've previously seen the GP before about your blood pressure which is high, and you've been taking amlodipine for this. You've also been told that your cholesterol is high, but so far you have been trying to address this through your diet. You have no allergies.

Your late father required an amputation in his sixties because he "had a bad blood supply".

You're finding it difficult to exercise but you do try to participate in a round of golf when you can. You have recently retired from your stock broking position. You have smoked for most of your life, but having previously smoked 30 a day for the past 30 years, you've managed to cut it down to about 4 or 5 a day. You enjoy a bottle of red wine with your wife every night and a glass of brandy with your colleagues at social functions.

If asked about your ideas, concerns and expectations please offer the information below
You are somewhat embarrassed that you cannot keep up with your colleagues and are concerned about your overall health, particularly despite your best efforts with regards to giving up smoking. You are keen to know if there's anything that can be done.

Mark Scheme: Leg Pain

Task:	Achieved	Not Achieved
Introduces himself / herself		
Confirms patient details and purpose of consultation		
Established the main presenting complaint		
Ascertains the site of the pain—and whether it is unilateral or bilateral		
Elicits the onset and duration of symptoms		
Ascertains the character and radiation of the pain		
Asks about worsening factors (i.e. exertion, pain at night or lying flat)		
Asks about relieving factors (i.e. rest, sitting or leaning forward)		
Asks about exercise tolerance		
Asks about associated symptoms—back pain, numbness, weakness, incontinence, change in colour or temperature		
Asks about past medical history specifically diabetes, hypertension, stroke, hypercholesterolaemia		
Asks about medications and allergies		
Asks about family history & social history including alcohol and smoking		
Plans to examine or asks for examination findings		
Summarises findings concisely		

Able to provide appropriate differential diagnoses Intermittent claudication secondary to peripheral vascular disease Spinal claudication Sciatica Deep vein thrombosis		
Suggests appropriate investigations Routine bloods - FBC -looking for anaemia, ESR underlying inflammatory process, fasting glucose, lipid levels ECG Imaging - Doppler ultrasonography (ABPI)		
Appropriate management plan & follow-up Offers lifestyle advice -smoking cessation, exercise, weight reduction Offers a review appointment to see how they are managing. Considers antiplatelet drugs, vasodilators If no improvement to suggest referral to vascular surgeons		
Acknowledges & addresses patient's ideas, concerns and expectations		
Gives patient opportunity to ask questions		
Examiner's global mark	/5	
Actor/helper's global mark	/5	
Total station mark	/30	

Learning Points

- The history is key in distinguishing behind the different causes of leg pain. The quick resolution of symptoms upon resting suggests a vascular cause and should be investigated as such, however you should be mindful of other differential diagnoses—including spinal stenosis (characteristically relieved by leaning forward), sciatica (which produces 'shooting' pains down the leg) and deep vein thrombosis (in the presence of risk factors for venous thromboembolism).

- 80% of patients' symptoms improve with a combination of medical treatment and modification of lifestyle factors, and these should be promoted in all cases of non-critical limb ischaemia.

- Remember that in the general practice setting, you will probably not have access to a Doppler, however you should be able to recognise when a chronic history of intermittent claudication becomes an ischaemic limb! Remember the *six P's:* pain, pallor, pulselessness, parasthesia, paralysis and poikilothermia (perishingly cold!). Do not delay—you might just save their limb.

Case 2: Lump in the groin

Candidate's Instructions

You are the foundation year doctor working in General Practice and have been asked to see a 47 year old gentleman Gary who has presented to the GP surgery complaining of a lump in his groin. Please take a full history.

After 6 minutes the examiner will stop you and ask you to summarise back your findings, suggest your differential diagnoses and your initial management plan.

Examiner's Instructions

A 47 year old gentleman Gary, has presented to the GP surgery complaining of a lump in his groin.

The candidate, is acting as the foundation year doctor Doctor, and has been asked to take a history from the patient.

After 6 minutes please stop the candidate at whatever stage they are and ask them to present the case with their primary differential diagnoses. Following this ask them what their next steps regarding investigations and management will be.
If they ask, give them the examination findings below:
Examination findings:
Gary is comfortable at rest. His observations are normal. His abdomen is soft and non tender, with no palpable masses felt. You examine his groin while he stands, he has a positive cough reflex on the left. It is reducible and soft. The skin around and on top of it is not red.
All other systemic examinations are normal.
Questions to ask if there is time:
What is the difference between a direct and indirect hernia?
What are the complications of hernias?

Actor's Instructions

You are a 47 year old gentleman, Gary, who has presented to the GP surgery complaining of a lump in his groin, which tracks down to your scrotum on the left.

ONLY OFFER INFORMATION IF SPECIFICALLY ASKED

You first noticed it when you came home after a particularly strenuous day at work a couple of months ago, when you were lifting a wheelbarrow of bricks. It was sore at the time however the pain has since subsided so you assumed it would go away by itself. However, since then you've been unfortunate enough to suffer from a particularly bad cold which has required you to take time off work—and over the last few days you've noticed the lump "popping out" when you had a coughing fit.

You can still push it back in, so it has not bothered you too much. Additionally, you've not had any pain aside from some mild discomfort, and your bowels have continued to work as normal though you admit to suffering from some constipation. You've not had any previous surgery. You've not noticed any changes in the skin overlying the lump.

You have no other medical history and you are not on any regular medications, however your GP did comment on the fact you're slightly overweight during your previous appointment.

You are a builder and do a lot of heavy lifting and manual labour. You do not smoke and drink a couple pints per week. You are married and live with your wife and kids at home.

If asked about your ideas, concerns and expectations please offer the information below
Your chief concern is that the swelling has become a bit more troublesome, and that it may require an operation. This would impact your ability to return to work, and you cannot afford to do so as you rely on your business as your source of income.

Mark Scheme: Lump in the groin

Task:	Achieved	Not Achieved
Introduces himself / herself		
Confirms patient details and purpose of consultation		
Established the main presenting complaint		
Ascertains the characteristics of the lump including the site and if it is unilateral/bilateral		
Asks about the onset of presentation and timing		
Asks if lump is tender or has changed over time		
Ascertains symptoms suggestive of incarceration: irreducibility, overlying skin changes, disturbance of bowel habit (absolute constipation, failure to pass flatus)		
Asks about previous surgery		
Asks about past medical history		
Asks about medications and allergies		
Asks about family history & social history including occupation, alcohol and smoking		
Plans to examine or asks for examination findings		
Summarises findings concisely		
Able to provide appropriate differential diagnoses Inguinal Hernia - direct or indirect Femoral hernia Incisional hernia Possible testicular lump		
Suggests appropriate investigations Usually a clinical diagnosis Can perform an ultrasound scan to confirm		
Offers lifestyle advice: Weight loss Increasing dietary fibre to avoid constipation Proper lifting techniques - manual handling course		
Appropriate management plan & follow-up Referral to surgeons for definitive treatment—mesh repair Offers a review appointment to see how they are managing.		
Acknowledges & addresses patient's ideas, concerns and expectations		

Safety net—emergency help to be sought if sudden onset pain, irreducibility, bowel disturbance, skin changes		
Gives patient opportunity to ask questions		
Examiner's global mark	/5	
Actor/helper's global mark	/5	
Total station mark	/30	

Learning points:

- Though the location of the lump and the history presented is highly suggestive of an inguinal hernia, it is still prudent to be mindful of the differential diagnosis of any lump that presents in the region. Examples include a hydrocele (which one could get above on palpation) or an abscess (seen particularly amongst intravenous drug users).
- The definitive management is operative, as hernias tend to worsen as time goes on. However, much can be done in the GP setting to counsel the patient about lifestyle factors that hasten the need for operative management. Preventing constipation, encouraging proper lifting techniques, and encouraging weight loss all contribute towards the prevention of hernia formation and reduce the risk of strangulation.
- Red flag symptoms—exquisite tenderness, irreducibility, failure to open bowels or pass flatus, overlying skin changes—suggest the incarceration of intestinal contents in the hernia and possible strangulation. These patients should be referred to hospital for urgent surgical assessment.

Case 3: Lump in the breast

Candidate's Instructions

You are the foundation year doctor working in General Practice and have been asked to see a 50 year old woman Sarah has presented to the GP surgery after having found a lump in her breast. Please take a full history.

After 6 minutes the examiner will stop you and ask you to summarise back your findings, suggest your differential diagnoses and your initial management plan.

Examiner's Instructions

A 50 year old woman Sarah has presented to the GP surgery after having found a lump in her breast.

The candidate, is acting as the foundation year doctor, and has been asked to take a history from the patient. After 6 minutes please stop the candidate at whatever stage they are and ask them to present the case with their primary differential diagnoses. Following this ask them what their next steps regarding investigations and management will be.

If they ask, give them the examination findings below:

Examination findings:

Sarah is comfortable at rest with normal observations. On examination of the breasts, there is some mild dimpling of the skin on the left with nipple inversion. There is a small hard fixed lump in the upper quadrant that seems slightly uncomfortable. All other systemic examinations are normal.

Questions to ask if there is time:

Where are the main sights of spread from breast cancer?

What types of breast cancer are there, and which have a worse prognosis?

Actor's instructions

You are a 50 year old woman Sarah, who has presented to the GP surgery after having found a lump in her breast.

ONLY OFFER INFORMATION IF SPECIFICALLY ASKED

You first noticed it about two months ago on the left upper side of the breast, whilst bathing. However, you did not think much of it at the time. It's not particularly painful but you think it's grown in size over the last two months, to about the size of a marble. It's quite hard in nature and it seems to be quite fixed. You've not noticed any discharge from the nipple, but you did notice a speck of blood on the inner surface of your bra the other day. The breast itself looks normal, with no skin or nipple changes. Your weight has been stable, you've not been in pain and as far as you know, you've not noticed any swellings elsewhere. You have not had any trauma to the area.

You've stopped having your periods about 18 months ago. You've not noticed any abnormal bleeding or discharge from down below. You're a mother of two children, aged 13 and 17, both of whom were born vaginally with no complications during pregnancy or childbirth. You don't have any medical problems, nor are you on any regular medications; though you've been experiencing some hot flushes recently and your GP believes this is down to the menopause, you've been reluctant to try HRT yet.

You don't smoke, but you do drink about 15 units of alcohol per week.

If asked about your ideas, concerns and expectations please offer the information below
However, your mother died of ovarian cancer in her 50s and you have read in the newspaper that there is a link between that and breast cancer—and you are worried that this may too be cancer.

Mark Scheme: Lump in the breast

Task:	Achieved	Not Achieved
Introduces himself / herself		
Confirms patient details and purpose of consultation		
Established the main presenting complaint		
Asks about the lump - size, site, shape		
Asks if the lump is painful, if it is mobile or fixed to the skin		
Ask about nipple changes - discharge or bleeding, or change in shape/inversion		
Asks about overlying skin changes (eg. peau d' orange)		
Asks about red flag symptoms - weight loss, loss of appetite, lethargy, night sweats, fevers		
Asks about bony pain or swelling elsewhere (e.g. lymph nodes)		
Asks about recent trauma and breastfeeding		
Asks about past medical history		
Asks about medications and allergies specifically about hormone replacement therapy		
Asks about family history of cancer & social history including alcohol and smoking		
Plans to examine or asks for examination findings		
Summarises findings concisely		
Able to provide appropriate differential diagnoses Breast carcinoma Duct Ectasia Cystic disease Benign mammary dysplasia		
Suggests appropriate investigations Triple assessment History and examination Imaging - mammography/USS Fine needle aspiration (biopsy)		
Appropriate management plan & follow-up 2 week wait referral to breast surgeons Offers a review appointment to see how they are managing.		

Acknowledges & addresses patient's ideas, concerns and expectations		
Gives patient opportunity to ask questions		
Examiner's global mark	/5	
Actor/helper's global mark	/5	
Total station mark	/30	

Learning Points

- Breast lumps are a cause for concern amongst women (and men) but fortunately, most are benign—caused by fibroadenomas. These typically present in younger women of childbearing age, with non-tender, highly mobile masses that come and go as related to hormonal changes in the body.

- The key things to look out for in the presentation that suggests malignancy include a hard/irregular lump, tethering to bone or skin, bloody discharge and lymphadenopathy. These patients should be referred under the "two week rule" to secondary care.

- In the general practice setting you should have a low threshold for referring patients of any age with a family history of breast or uterine cancer, due to its potential heritability (with mutations of the BRCA1/2 tumour suppressor genes).

Chapter 6: Renal & Urology

Case 1: Lower urinary tract symptoms

Candidate's Instructions:

You are the foundation year doctor working in General Practice and have been asked to see a 55 year old woman Geeta who has presented to the GP surgery complaining of feeling unwell. Take a full history and address their ideas, concerns and expectations.

After 6 minutes the examiner will stop you and ask you to summarise back your findings, suggest your differential diagnoses and your initial management plan.

Examiner's Instructions:

A 55 year old woman Geeta has presented to the GP surgery complaining of feeling unwell.

The candidate, is acting as the foundation year doctor, and has been asked to take a brief history from the patient.

After 6 minutes please stop the candidate and ask them to present the case and propose their next steps regarding investigations and management.

If they ask, give them the examination findings below:
Examination findings:
Geeta is comfortable at rest, with normal observations. Her abdomen is soft and she has mild suprapubic tenderness. Her urine dip result with her that she just performed with the nurse. It is positive for moderate nitrites and leucocytes. There is no blood present.

All other systemic examinations are normal.

Actor's Instructions:

A 55 year old woman Geeta has presented to the GP surgery complaining of feeling unwell.

ONLY OFFER INFORMATION IF SPECIFICALLY ASKED

When the consultation begins explain that you have just done a urine dip test with the nurse who has given you the following results to take to the doctor.

Nitrites moderate
Leucocytes moderate
Blood negative

For the last 3 days it has been painful when you pass urine, it is a burning sensation. I have been going to pass urine more often and have had to rush to get there on time. You have not had any incontinence. You have not noticed any blood in your urine. You have not had any fevers. You have also had some lower tummy pain that is a mild ache from time to time.

You have high blood pressure but no other past medical history. You have only had one previous urinary tract infection in your twenties. As far as you know you do not have any renal tract abnormalities and have normal functioning kidneys.

You live with your husband and are not sexually active. You have not had a recent sexual health screen but feel you are not at risk of a sexually transmitted infection. You have not had any abnormal vaginal discharge or bleeding. You do not smoke and do not drink. You are a housewife.

The candidate will now have a discussion with the examiner. Following this they will take some time to address your ideas, concerns and expectations. You have some specific questions:

1. Ask the doctor what your symptoms could be attributed to, as you thought it may be a urinary tract infection.

2. You have been doing some reading of your daughters medical textbooks, as she is studying medicine currently and you had some questions about your condition. Ask them to explain what a recurrent UTI is, and ask what the difference between a relapse and a reinfection. You are wondering if you fall into the category of recurrent UTI? Because you would like a kidney scan as you are worried.

3. The nurses always ask me to do a mid-stream urine, but no one has told me how to do this, could you explain.

Mark Scheme: Lower Urinary Tract Infection

Task:	Achieved	Not Achieved
Introduces himself / herself		
Confirms patient details and purpose of consultation		
Established the main presenting complaint		
Asks specifically about the nature of her pain, frequency and urgency, haematuria.		
Asks if she has had any fevers or loin pain		
Sensitively screens for a sexually transmitted infection.		
Asks about her past medical history including previous urinary tract infections		
Ask if she or any family members have any renal tract abnormalities or known impaired renal function.		
Asks about medications, allergies and social history including alcohol and smoking		
Plans to examine or asks for examination findings		
Summarises findings concisely		
Able to provide appropriate differential diagnoses Likely urinary tract infection Exclude pyelonephritis		
Suggests appropriate investigations Urine dip and culture		
Appropriate management plan & follow-up Antibiotics therapy according to guidelines - trimethoprim or nitrofurantoin. Suitable pain relief with paracetamol Offers a review appointment to see how they are managing.		
Acknowledges & addresses patient's ideas, concerns and expectations		
Gives patient opportunity to ask questions		
Explains diagnosis and management to the patient.		
Provides safety netting advice to return if she develops a fever or loin pain or if her symptoms do not improve.		

Addresses the complex questions that the patient has and suggests alternative to medical textbook, patient friendly resources.		
Explains clearly to the patient how to take a mid-stream urine.		
Examiner's Global Mark	/5	
Actor / Helper's Global Mark	/5	
Total Station Mark	/30	

Learning Points

- A recurrent UTI refers to 2 or more infections in 6 months or 3 or more infections in 1 year. A recurrent UTI can either be due to relapse or reinfection. Relapse is a recurrent UTI with the same strain of organism. Relapse is a likely cause if infection recurs shortly after treatment. Reinfection is a recurrent UTI with a different strain or species of organism. It is the likely cause of recurrent infection more than two weeks after the initial treatment.

- It is important to clearly explain to a patient how to take a mid-stream urine: Firstly the peri-urethral area should be cleaned. About 10ml of urine should be collected at mid-stream- the middle point of urination, without interrupting urine flow to start or stop the collection. It must be collected into a sterile container.

- Patients will often come into your consultation room and know what is wrong with them, listen to what their thoughts are and work together with them to build a rapport. Some patients will do excessive research but find it difficult to understand or interpret their research, point them in the right direction for resources more suited for their understanding.

Case 2: Haematuria

Candidate's Instructions

You are the foundation year doctor working in General Practice and have been asked to see a 64 year old gentleman Winston who has presented to the GP surgery complaining of blood in his urine. Please take a full history.

After 6 minutes the examiner will stop you and ask you to summarise back your findings, suggest your differential diagnoses and your initial management plan.

Examiner's Instructions

A 64 year old gentleman Winston has presented to the GP surgery complaining of blood in his urine.

The candidate, is acting as the foundation year doctor, and has been asked to take a history from the patient.

After 6 minutes please stop the candidate and ask them to present the case with their primary differential diagnoses. Following this ask them what their next steps regarding investigations and management will be.

If they ask, give them the examination findings below:
Examination findings:
Winston is comfortable at rest, does look very slim. His abdomen is soft and non tender, with no palpable bladder. Urine dip shows 4+ blood and is a rose colour.
All other systemic examinations are normal.
Questions to ask if there is time:
What is the TNM staging for bladder cancer and how does that affect the treatment given?

Actor's instructions

You are a 64 year old gentleman Winston who has presented to the GP surgery complaining of blood in his urine

ONLY OFFER INFORMATION IF SPECIFICALLY ASKED

It's bright red in colour, and painless. It's been troubling you for the past week, within which you've noticed it becoming more and more frequent. You've also noticed you've been having more of an urge to urinate recently. You haven't had any abdominal pain, no burning or stinging when you pass urine, no discharge from the penis, nor have you had any fever.

You've not had any falls or otherwise any trauma that might have otherwise explained the bleeding. However you have been feeling a bit run down recently, and you've been having to stop to catch your breath when climbing the stairs. You think you've lost a bit of weight, as your shirts do not fit as they once did.
You're otherwise well, you have high blood pressure which is controlled by tablets but have not had any major illnesses in the past. You have been a lifelong smoker (20 a day since childhood) and you've found it difficult to give up. You have the occasional pint.

You are a semi-retired decorator. Your family have all been well, but your father who used to run the decorating family business, had some bladder problems late in his life.
If asked about your ideas, concerns and expectations please offer the information below
You're worried about whether you're going to need a catheter because of the bleeding. You remember having had to care for your father who suffered from infections and blockages of the catheter and you think you would struggle to cope with one.

Mark Scheme: Haematuria

Task:	Achieved	Not Achieved
Introduces himself / herself		
Confirms patient details and purpose of consultation		
Established the main presenting complaint		
Asks about nature of haematuria: duration, intermittent or continuous and progression		
- Asks about the blood - colour (fresh red, dark) and amount of bleeding.		
Asks about red flag symptoms - weight loss, loss of appetite, lethargy, night sweats, fevers		
- Asks about symptoms of anaemia—tiredness, breathlessness		
- Lower Urinary Tract Symptoms associated with storage (volume, urgency, frequency, nocturia)		
- Lower Urinary Tract Symptoms associated with voiding (terminal dribbling, poor flow, hesitancy, sensation of incomplete voiding)		
- Lower Urinary Tract Symptoms associated with infection (dysuria)		
Asks about past medical history		
Asks about medications and allergies		
Asks about family history & social history including occupation, alcohol and smoking		
Plans to examine or asks for examination findings		

Summarises findings concisely		
Able to provide appropriate differential diagnoses Bladder transitional cell carcinoma Other malignancies of the renal tract Urinary tract infection Glomerulonephritis Prostate cancer / BPH Drug reaction e.g. rifampicin,		
Suggests appropriate investigations Routine Bloods - FBC to look for anaemia, renal function tests and electrolytes, PSA Urine tests (dipstick, cytology) Imaging - Cystoscopy + biopsy + CT		
Appropriate management plan & follow-up 2 week wait referral to urology Offers a review appointment to see how they are managing.		
Acknowledges & addresses patient's ideas, concerns and expectations		
Gives patient opportunity to ask questions		
Examiner's global mark	/5	
Actor/helper's global mark	/5	
Total station mark	/35	

Learning Points

- In the general practice setting, anybody over the age of forty-five years with visible haematuria, or over sixty with microscopic haematuria, in the absence of a urinary tract infection, should be referred for urgent urological assessment to rule out cancer.

- Risk factors for bladder cancer in the Western world revolve around the exposure to polycyclic aromatic hydrocarbons—in other words, tobacco smokers, and those with occupational exposure (industrial workers in regular contact with metalwork, paint, petroleum, dyes and solvents).

- Operative management of bladder cancer, or complications from the cancer itself (e.g. clot retention) can necessitate the use of a catheter, which can cause a patient distress, embarrassment or inconvenience—particularly on day to day life when used long term. Be mindful of this when counselling your patients!

Chapter 7: Endocrinology, Dermatology & Musculoskeletal

Case 1: Diabetic Management

Candidate's instructions

You are the foundation year doctor working in General Practice and have been asked to see a 42 year old gentleman Praveen who has attended the GP surgery for a routine diabetic follow up but he is complaining of feeling funny in the last few weeks. Please take a full history.

After 6 minutes the examiner will stop you and ask you to summarise back your findings, suggest your differential diagnoses and your initial management plan.

Examiner's instructions:

A 42 year old gentleman Praveen has attended the GP surgery for a routine diabetic follow up but he is complaining of feeling funny in the last few weeks.

The candidate, is acting as the foundation year doctor, and has been asked to take a history from the patient.

After 6 minutes please stop the candidate at whatever stage they are and ask them to present the case with their primary differential diagnoses. Following this ask them what their next steps regarding investigations and management will be.

If they ask, give them the examination findings below:
Examination findings:
Praveen is comfortable, current BM 7.8. Observations are normal. All other systemic examinations are normal.

Results:
HbA1c has been stable – last performed 4 months ago 42mmolmol (7.0%)

Questions to ask if there is time:
How is a formal diagnosis of Type 2 Diabetes made?
What are the complications of diabetes?

Actor's instructions

You are a 42 year old gentleman Praveen who has attended the GP surgery for a routine diabetic follow up but he is complaining of feeling funny in the last few weeks.

ONLY OFFER INFORMATION IF SPECIFICALLY ASKED

You were diagnosed with Type 2 diabetes 2 years ago and have been on Metformin and Gliclazide, which was added 8 months ago. Your past medical history includes asthma which is well controlled with Salbutamol inhalers alone. You smoke 10/day and drink 4-5 pints on the weekends with friends.

Every 3-4 months, you have a blood test done at the GP practice to check your diabetes control is satisfactory. The last test was within range so there were no changes to medication. You have annual checks for your eyes at the hospital. The GP also checks your blood pressure, feet, urine and blood test on regular intervals. You believe some of this for monitoring your heart, nerves and kidneys.

Unfortunately your diet has slipped lately due to being too busy to cook, so you have probably not had as great control as previously and you used to go on long walks and jogs, but due to work being more busy, you have been too tired.

Until the last 3 weeks, you were well but have recently noticed that you are increasingly having episodes where you feel faint and dizzy. This is accompanied with sweating and sometimes palpitations. You have not been worried much as eating seems to help these symptoms and so decided not to seek advice until today.

You were a builder but have recently been offered a job as an HGV driver which you intend to take up in the next few weeks. You do not drink alcohol and do not smoke.

Your family history includes both parents with diabetes. You have no allergies.

If asked about your ideas, concerns and expectations please offer the information below

You are quite happy with the current medications and do not want to make any changes to them. You are adamant they are fine, but if your doctor explains why it is dangerous for you to stay on Gliclazide as you are about to be an HGV driver and why the change in necessary, you understand and accept this. You then agree to try the new medication.

Mark Scheme: Diabetic Management

Task:	Achieved	Not Achieved
Introduces himself / herself		
Confirms patient details and purpose of consultation		
Established the main presenting complaint		
Elicits duration of current management		
Asks about current monitoring : BP, Urine, Feet, Eyes		
Asks about last HbA1c result, date of test and interprets correctly		
Asks about past medical history specifically Ischaemic heart disease/heart failure , osteoporosis, bladder Ca (ie risks of glitazones), renal failure, stroke		
Asks about medications and allergies		
Asks about family history & social history including alcohol and smoking		
Asks about diet and exercise		
Elicits symptoms of Hypoglycaemia - dizziness, sweating, improved with eating		
Safety net for Hypoglycaemia in future (patient leaflet) considering occupation.		
Checks understanding		
Plans to examine or asks for examination findings		
Summarises findings concisely		

Able to provide appropriate differential diagnoses Hypoglycaemia secondary to gliclazide		
Suggests appropriate investigations Routine Bloods -HbA1c in 3-4 months Urine for dipstick and/or Albumin:Creatinine ratio Examining the feet and eye tests annually.		
Appropriate management plan & follow-up Switching Gliclazide to alternative therapy Provides appropriate alternate agent – glitazone/gliptin. Insulin NOT an option. Offers a review appointment to see how they are managing.		
Acknowledges & addresses patient's ideas, concerns and expectations		
Gives patient opportunity to ask questions		
Examiner's Global Mark	/5	
Actor / Helper's Global Mark	/5	
Total Station Mark	/30	

Learning points

- Sulphonylureas such as Gliclazide are known to cause Hypoglycaemia, which is highly significant in this scenario as the patient is about to drive HGVs which can predispose not only him but also others on the road to accidents.

- Patients often have concerns when their established medical regime requires change. Elicit and address their concerns and explain to them why the change is necessary. If at all possible never change multiple drugs at the same time as this can lead to confusion and errors and make interpretation of approval or deterioration difficult for the clinician.

- Be aware of the adverse effects of common medications such as Metformin, Gliclazide, Pioglitazone and Insulin.

Case 2: Tired all the time

Candidate's Instructions

You are the foundation year doctor working in General Practice and have been asked to see a 40 year old lady Hettie who has presented to the GP surgery complaining of being "tired all the time". Please take a full history and perfomr a focused examination.

After 6 minutes the examiner will stop you and ask you to summarise back your findings, suggest your differential diagnoses and your initial management plan.

Examiner's instructions

A 40 year old lady Hettie has presented to the GP surgery complaining of being "tired all the time".

The candidate, is acting as the foundation year doctor, and has been asked to take a history from the patient. If they get the wrong examination, prompt them to perform a thyroid examination.

After six minutes ask them to present the case with their primary differential diagnoses and ask them what their next steps regarding investigations and management will be.

Questions to ask if there is time:
What are the causes of Hypothyroidism?

Actor's instructions

You are a 40 year old lady Hettie who has presented to the GP surgery complaining of being "tired all the time"

ONLY OFFER INFORMATION IF SPECIFICALLY ASKED

You have come to the GP practice today as you have been feeling increasingly tired for the last 6-8 months. You have had good appetite and have been able to sleep well, with good levels of concentration. Your mood has not been any different and you are enjoying your hobbies of cycling and painting as usual. You have not travelled in the last 12 months.

You have not had shortness of breath, chest pain, palpitations, loss of consciousness or any changes in your urinary habits.

There have been no rashes, joint pains, fevers, night sweats or weight loss.

Your weight has in fact been very difficult to lose as you have been trying for nearly 2 years. You have also noticed that you find you need a jacket even during the summer. Your bowel motions have been sluggish and your menstrual periods have been particularly heavy during this time.

Your family history includes Mum who has underactive thyroid and Dad who has Type 1 diabetes.

You have no other medical problems, you are not on any regular medications and have no drug allergies. You are an accountant, with 2 kids and a husband at home and you have never smoked and drink 1-2 glasses of wine on the weekends.

If asked about your ideas, concerns and expectations please offer the information below
You are mostly concerned about being so tired that you can not carry out your daily tasks at work and then look after the kids at home. You fall asleep while trying to help them with homework.

Mark Scheme: Tired all the Time

Task:	Achieved	Not Achieved
Introduces himself / herself		
Confirms patient details and purpose of consultation		
Established the main presenting complaint		
Assess cardiovascular symptoms: Shortness of breath, chest pain, palpitations, loss of consciousness		
Assesses psychiatric symptoms: mood, appetite, concentration		
Assesses thyroid status: cold/heat intolerance, diarrhea/constipation, hair loss		
Assesses rheumatological symptoms: joint pains, rashes, haematuria		
Asks about red flag symptoms - weight loss, loss of appetite, lethargy, night sweats, fevers		
Examines the relevant system: Thyroid		
Hands & Nails: warm/sweaty/cold/palmar erythema/tremor & onycholysis/acropachy		
Pulse: Tachycardia/bradycardia/AF		
Eyes: loss of outer 1/3rd/ Chemosis/ Lid lag/ Ophthalmoplegia/ Exophthalmos (stand behind and look from above)		
Neck: presence of lump and it's site, size, shape and colour, temperature, tenderness, mobility, consistency, nodularity and surface		

Palpation of lump when swallowing and tongue out		
Summarises findings concisely		
Able to provide appropriate differential diagnoses Hypothyroidism Anaemia Diabetes		
Suggests appropriate investigations Routine bloods - FBC - anaemia, Thyroid function -T4, TSH, HbA1c Blood glucose ECG		
Appropriate management plan & follow-up Offers a review appointment to see how they are managing and for review of blood tests If hypothyroid may need to consider treatment with thyroxine If anaemic consider type of anaemia and treatment accordingly		
Acknowledges & addresses patient's ideas, concerns and expectations		
Gives patient opportunity to ask questions		
Examiner's Global Mark	/5	
Actor / Helper's Global Mark	/5	
Total Station Mark	/30	

Learning points

- A large number of causes can present with tiredness in the GP setting. It is important to keep an open mind and have a structured approach to your history taking. Most importantly, look for features suggesting conditions that are common such as thyroid disease and those that are malignant.

- When assessing thyroid status, in addition to assessing the goitre, remember to assess for peripheral manifestations such as pulse, thyroid eye disease and nail changes. In addition you can assess reflexes and peripheral myopathy.

- As there is limited time in a GP setting, remember to take a concise history and tailor your examination towards it, whilst ensuring you have ruled out the red flags such as weight loss early in the consultation.

Case 3: Skin Rash

Candidate's Instructions

You are the foundation year doctor working in General Practice and have been asked to see a 38 year old gentleman Spencer who has presented to the GP surgery with a rash. The rash is seen on both elbows on the flexors surfaces and is raised with dry scaly plaques. Please take a full history and perform a brief examination.

After 6 minutes the examiner will stop you and ask you to summarise back your findings, suggest your differential diagnoses and your initial management plan.

Examiner's instructions

A 38 year old gentleman Spencer has presented to the GP surgery with a rash that is seen on both elbows on the flexors surfaces and is raised with dry scaly plaques, in keeping with active psoriasis.

The candidate, is acting as the foundation year doctor and has been asked to take a history and examine the patient.

After 6 minutes please stop the candidate and ask them to present the case with their primary differential diagnoses. Following this ask them what their next steps regarding investigations and management will be.

Actor's instructions

You are a 38 year old gentleman Spencer who has presented to the GP surgery with a persistent red rash on both elbows for the last 6 years which has not grown in size.

ONLY OFFER INFORMATION IF SPECIFICALLY ASKED

You have noticed that the rash is quite thick, appears red although it is not painful, has not bled or oozed pus. There are no blisters and you don't have other rashes on the body. The rash sometimes reduces after you have worked in the summer when it's sunny. You think it often becomes worse when you are stressed.

You tried some moisturisers last year for this rash but they seemed to have hardly had any effect. You had left it then but now, as you will be attending your friend's wedding in 4 weeks, you want to get rid of it as it is extremely embarrassing.

You have had no fevers, joint pains, swellings, night sweats, weight loss or change in appetite. You have no ulcers in your mouth, have good bowel movement and no changes in your urinary habits.

You have previously had your appendix removed, but otherwise have been healthy. You have not been travelling in the last 3 years. You do not take any regular medications and you are only allergic to hazelnuts.

You have been a builder for the last 20 years, live with your wife and son aged 6, have no pets, smoke 15 a day and drink 2-3 pints of alcohol with friends every night after work.

You had an uncle who had a similar rash called psoriasis, but he had it more widespread and he always complained of pain in his joints. There is no other family history of rashes.

If asked about your ideas, concerns and expectations please offer the information below

A few weeks ago, you heard of a new drug called Methotrexate which you can take tablets of and is known to be very effective at controlling this type of rash. You are highly keen on taking it so that you can be free of it by the wedding. As it is a new drug, you believe it is also quite safe to take and want to try it.

You don't understand why the doctor is not happy to prescribe it — you ask if it is because it's expensive. It is only when they explain that it can potentially cause failure of production of blood and the immune system, cause lung and liver damage that you appreciate the risks and agree on trying a different treatment instead.

Mark Scheme: Skin Rash

Task:	Achieved	Not Achieved
Introduces himself / herself		
Confirms patient details and purpose of consultation		
Established the main presenting complaint		
Asks about duration, evolution (growth, itching, pain, any bleeding or pus), any other lesions on body		
Assesses relieving factors (sunshine, creams), exacerbating factors (smoking, alcohol, stress, trauma, drugs)		
Assesses joint pain, swelling, stiffness, oral ulcers, bowel motions, urinary habits and recent infections		
Asks about red flag symptoms - weight loss, loss of appetite, lethargy, night sweats, fevers		
Asks about past medical history, medications and allergies		
Asks about family history & social history including alcohol and smoking		
Atopy: hayfever, asthma, allergies, eczema		
Plans to examine or asks for examination findings		
Examines rash: site, size, shape, colour, described as a plaque		

Assesses demarcation (well defined vs poor), temperature, tenderness, blood/pus, blister formation		
Asks to pain/stiffness/ range of motion in joint and other areas of the body for similar rashes - hands/ears		
Summarises findings concisely		
Able to provide appropriate differential diagnoses • Psoriasis • Dermatitis/eczema • Lichen Planus • Discoid Lupus		
Appropriate management plan & follow-up • Starts a weak steroid cream / Vitamin D analogue or combination • Offers a review appointment to see how they are managing.		
Acknowledges & addresses patient's ideas, concerns and expectations		
Explains why Methotrexate is not appropriate at this stage (Side effects: neutropenia, pulmonary fibrosis, cirrhosis)		
Gives patient opportunity to ask questions		
Examiner's Global Mark	/5	
Actor / Helper's Global Mark	/5	
Total Station Mark	/30	

Learning points

- Remember the classic exacerbating and relieving factors of Psoriasis as in this scenario as it can greatly aid in the diagnosis of the rash.

- Know the stages of management of Psoriasis (emollients, steroid cream, vitamin D analogues, UV therapy, systemic agents like Methotrexate) and the common adverse effects of Methotrexate.

- The patient may already have an agenda of their own and want a specific treatment. It is only after finding out why they want it and addressing their concerns with full explanations that you will be able to reassure them.

Case 4: Skin Moles

Candidate's Instructions

You are the foundation year doctor working in General Practice and have been asked to see a 59 year old gentleman Hugo who has presented to the GP surgery with a small mole.
Please take a full history.

After 6 minutes the examiner will stop you and ask you to summarise back your findings, suggest your differential diagnoses and your initial management plan.

Examiner's instructions:

A 59 year old gentleman, Mr Hugo, has presented to the GP surgery with a small mole. It has a dark central raised region with a lighter irregular border that appears itchy with some evidence of bleeding.

The candidate, is acting as the foundation year doctor, and has been asked to take a history from the patient.

After 6 minutes please stop the candidate at whatever stage they are and ask them to present the case with their primary differential diagnoses. Following this ask them what their next steps regarding investigations and management will be.

Questions to ask if there is time:

What are the different types of skin cancers, how do they present differently?

What are the different type of treatment for skin cancer?

Actor's instructions

You are Hugo a 59 year old who has presented to the GP with a small mole, which your wife noticed on your back 2 weeks ago

ONLY OFFER INFORMATION IF SPECIFICALLY ASKED

The mole started bleeding yesterday and she commented that it had doubled in size during this time. It does not hurt, but you find it is itchy sometimes.

You enjoy travelling, both as part of work and leisure and have spent a significant part of your life away from the country, largely in the Mediterranean countries, Southeast Asia and South America. During your trips, you often go to the beach or seek spots where you can sunbathe. You don't use sunbeds and have not really been consistent with using any suncreams. Your skin does burn sometimes.

Your past medical history includes Type 2 diabetes for which you take Metformin, but otherwise you have been well.

You are a landscape photographer so spend a lot of time outside. You smoke 20 cigarettes a day and drink 3-4 pints 2-3 times a week. You live with your wife and a pet dog. You do not have any allergies.

Your Dad had skin cancer when he was in his 60s but recovered from it after some procedure and your mother had breast cancer when she was in her 50s.

If asked about your ideas, concerns and expectations please offer the information below

You are not particularly worried that it is something bad— it just looks like a mole when you looked at it in the mirror but have come as your wife was worried about it. You would rather not bother the doctor with something like this and are not particularly keen on going to the hospital as you have never liked going to one, but if the doctor explains why he thinks you need to go see the hospital doctors, you understand his reasoning and agree to it.

Mark Scheme: Skin mole

Task:	Achieved	Not Achieved
Introduces himself / herself		
Confirms patient details and purpose of consultation		
Established the main presenting complaint		
Asks about duration, evolution (growth, itching, pain, any bleeding or pus), any other lesions on body		
Assesses risk factors for sun exposure: travel abroad, sunbathing, use of sun bed, use of protective sun creams		
Asks about red flag symptoms - weight loss, loss of appetite, lethargy, night sweats, fevers		
Asks about past medical history		
Asks about medications and allergies		
Asks about family history & social history including alcohol and smoking		
Plans to examine or asks for examination findings		
Examines mole: site, size, shape, colour/pigmentation		
Assesses ABCDE (asymmetry, border, colour, diameter, evolution)		
Assesses demarcation (well defined vs poor), temperature, tenderness, blood/pus, blister formation		
Asks to examine lymph nodes and other areas of the body for similar moles.		

Summarises findings concisely		
Able to provide appropriate differential diagnoses • Malignant melanoma • Basal cell carcinoma • Squamous cell carcinoma • Benign melanocytic lesion		
Suggests appropriate investigations • Clinical diagnosis, however is sent for biopsy following excision		
Appropriate management plan & follow-up • Monitoring lesion (photos/measuring) • Urgent 2 week wait referral to Dermatology services • Offers a review appointment to see how they are managing.		
Acknowledges & addresses patient's ideas, concerns and expectations		
Gives patient opportunity to ask questions		
Examiner's Global Mark	/5	
Actor / Helper's Global Mark	/5	
Total Station Mark	/30	

Learning points

- Always remember to assess pigmented lesions with a suspicion of a possible Malignant Melanoma and use the ABCDE approach: A – asymmetry, B – border (even/uneven), C- colour (uniform or not), D – diameter (greater than 6mm), E – evolution (change of lesion over time/bleeding).

- It is vital to ask about sun exposure and family history in this scenario and any lesion with a suspected malignant nature such as Squamous cell carcinoma of the skin.

- Not everyone is concerned about a "mole" and it is important to explain the reason behind actions such as 2 week wait referral to ensure they follow this through and receive appropriate treatment.

Case 5: Back Pain

Candidate's Instructions

You are the foundation year doctor working in General Practice and have been asked to see a 30 year old gentleman Robert who has presented to the GP surgery complaining of back pain. Please take a full history.

After 6 minutes the examiner will stop you and ask you to summarise back your findings, suggest your differential diagnoses and your initial management plan.

Examiner Instructions

A 30 year old gentleman Robert has presented to the GP surgery complaining of back pain.

The candidate, is acting as the foundation year doctor, and has been asked to take a history from the patient.
After 6 minutes please stop the candidate and ask them to present the case with their primary differential diagnoses. Following this ask them what their next steps regarding investigations and management will be.
If they ask, give them the examination findings below:
Examination findings:
Robert is comfortable at rest, observations are normal. There are no visible deformities, tenderness over the lower lumbar spine, forward flexion and lateral flexion to right is limited by pain, positive straight leg raise on the right, numbness along lateral aspect of right foot, reduced ankle jerk on the right. All other systemic examinations are normal.

Questions to ask if there is time:
What is cauda equina and why is it an emergency?

Actor Instructions

You are a 30 year old gentleman Robert who has presented to the GP surgery complaining of back pain.

ONLY OFFER INFORMATION IF SPECIFICALLY ASKED

Two days ago you bent over to pick up a heavy bag of cement mix without bending your knees. As you stood up you suddenly felt a pain in your lower back that made you drop the cement.

At onset the pain was sharp and sudden but is now a constant ache. You have had back pain at work before but nothing like this. You were unable to continue working that day and have not worked since. Most movement makes the pain worse but you feel it most when you straighten your back or lean to the right side. Movement often triggers shooting pains down your right leg to the outside of your foot. You have pins and needles along the outside of your right foot.

You have not noticed any weakness, numbness or pins and needles elsewhere on your legs or genital area. You have full control of your bladder and bowels.

You have no other known health problems and you are feeling otherwise well. No fever, sweats or weight loss. You do not take any medications. You have been taking over the counter paracetamol but this is barely touching the pain. You have no drug allergies.

You are a construction worker. You drink about ten pints of beer at weekends and smoke ten cigarettes per day. You have a wife and child at home.

If asked about your ideas, concerns and expectations please offer the information below

You are very anxious about whether whatever is causing your back pain will interfere with your work as you are the sole income for your family and you have a young child to support. You want some kind of scan to confirm the diagnosis. You are very keen for a quick resolution to this problem and want whatever treatment is necessary as soon as possible.

You may become quite pushy in trying to get what you want if you do not feel satisfied with the plan but you calm down if the doctor acknowledges your frustration, explains their reasoning and handles the discussion professionally.

Mark Scheme: Back Pain

Task:	Achieved	Not Achieved
Introduces himself / herself		
Confirms patient details and purpose of consultation		
Established the main presenting complaint		
Asks about the pain - site, onset, character, radiation, associated symptoms and exacerbating factors.		
Asks about neuropathic pains down legs		
Asks about focal neurological features in the legs - weakness, numbness, paraesthesia		
Asks specifically about saddle anaesthesia and loss of sphincter control		
Asks about systemic features of malignancy / infection- loss of appetite, weight loss, fevers, night sweats		
Establishes what treatment patient has already enacted		
Asks about past medical history specifically previous trauma		
Asks about medications and allergies		
Asks about family history & social history including alcohol and smoking		
Plans to examine or asks for examination findings		
Summarises findings concisely		
Able to provide appropriate differential diagnoses		

Prolapsed inter-vertebral disc at L5/S1 level Sciatica Musculoskeletal back pain Exclude cauda equina		
Suggests appropriate investigations Clinical diagnosis no investigations necessary If pain does not resolve may consider an MRI If high risk of cauda equina - needs to be blue lighted to A&E for urgent MRI.		
Appropriate management plan & follow-up Simple analgesia (paracetamol +/- NSAID then follow WHO ladder) Gentle physical activity including prescribed back exercises, no strenuous activity Offers a review appointment to see how they are managing. Discuss criteria for referral to orthopaedics / physiotherapy / specialist lower back pain service		
Clear advice to return immediately in case of any red flag symptoms - saddle anaesthesia and loss of sphincter control, weakness.		
Acknowledges & addresses patient's ideas, concerns and expectations		
Gives patient opportunity to ask questions		
Examiner's Global Mark	/5	
Actor / Helper's Global Mark	/5	
Total Station Mark	/30	

Learning points

- It is essential to know and make a point of excluding red flag symptoms for back pain. You should also educate the patient to watch out for them. Key red flags include:

  - Previous history malignancy (however long ago)
  - Age 16< or >50 with NEW onset pain
  - Weight loss (unexplained)
  - Non-mechanical pain (worse at rest)
  - Thoracic pain
  - Previous longstanding steroid use
  - Saddle anaesthesia
  - Reduced anal tone
  - Urinary retention

- It is important to be aware of the guidelines on imaging and referral for physiotherapy and specialist assessment. It also helps to be aware of how long it realistically takes to see, for example, a physiotherapist in the community following referral.

- This station is as much about communication skills as it is about diagnostics. It is important that you build rapport, establish his social circumstances and elicit his concerns about the diagnosis and prognosis. This will enable you to address his concerns and calm or even pre-empt any discord over the management plan

Case 6: Acutely painful knee

Candidate's Instructions

You are the foundation year doctor working in General Practice and have been asked to see Ronan a 55 year old gentleman, has presented to the GP surgery complaining of a painful knee. Please take a full history.

After 6 minutes the examiner will stop you and ask you to summarise back your findings, suggest your differential diagnoses and your initial management plan.

Examiner's Instructions

Ronan a 55 year old gentleman, has presented to the GP surgery complaining of a painful knee.

The candidate, is acting as the foundation year doctor, and has been asked to take a history from the patient.

After 6 minutes please stop the candidate and ask them to present the case with their primary differential diagnoses. Following this ask them what their next steps regarding investigations and management will be.

If they ask, give them the examination findings below:
Examination findings:
Ronan is apyrexial and systemically well. The knee is erythematous and warm with a mild effusion and is tender to touch. Pain causes only mild restriction of range of movement. All other systemic examinations are normal.

Questions to ask if there is time:
What medication would you NOT give in an acute gout situation?

Actor's Instructions

You are Ronan a 55 year old gentleman, who has presented to the GP surgery complaining of a painful knee.

ONLY OFFER INFORMATION IF SPECIFICALLY ASKED

You have had severe pain in your right knee, which has been red and swollen, for the past 3 days. The pain is causing you to limp. The pain started 3 days ago and got gradually worse over the first 24 hours. At its worst it is 8 or 9 out of 10. It does not radiate. You find keeping the leg still and keeping weight off it helps. The knee has felt constantly stiff and swollen since the first day. You have not injured the knee and have not sustained any cuts that broke the skin around the knee. You have not had any recent trauma or surgery.

You have not had any symptoms of an infection recently (e.g. cough, cold, sore throat, rash, red eyes, painful urination, diarrhoea or vomiting). You have not been feeling feverish. You have never had anything like this before. You do not have similar symptoms in any other joints. You have not seen any growths or swellings on the skin around your joints.

You have high blood pressure and high cholesterol. You have also been told that you are overweight. You take amlodipine, bendroflumethiazide and atorvastatin. You have no allergies. You think your father had similar symptoms but can't remember what caused the symptoms. He also had kidney stones.

You are an investment banker. You live with your wife and three children. You have a rich diet including lots of meat and shellfish. You tend to drink little water, averaging about a pint per day. You do not smoke. You drink 10-15 pints of beer per week. It was your son's wedding last weekend so you drank a lot more than usual.

If asked about your ideas, concerns and expectations please offer the information below
The pain is interfering with your ability to concentrate at work. You are concerned that this might happen again and hope that the doctor can prevent recurrence.

Mark Scheme: Acutely Swollen Knee

Task:	Achieved	Not Achieved
Introduces himself / herself		
Confirms patient details and purpose of consultation		
Established the main presenting complaint		
Asks about the pain - site, onset, character, radiation, associated symptoms and exacerbating factors.		
Establishes timeline - speed of onset, duration, precedence		
Asks about associated features- redness, swelling, stiffness		
Asks about possible triggers for pain- trauma, infection, alcohol		
Asks about distribution of symptoms and whether any other joints are affected		
Asks about systemic features of malignancy / infection- loss of appetite, weight loss, fevers, night sweats, rash		
Asks about past medical history specifically osteoarthritis, rheumatoid arthritis, psoriasis, gout		
Asks about past surgical history specifically previous operations on the knee		
Asks about medications and allergies		
Asks about family history & social history including diet, alcohol and smoking		
Plans to examine or asks for examination findings		

Summarises findings concisely		
Able to provide appropriate differential diagnoses Gout Septic Arthritis Fracture secondary to trauma		
Suggests appropriate investigations Routine Bloods - inflammatory markers to exclude infection, Urate, Renal function. Imaging - Xray/CT/MRI to exclude osteomyelitis, septic arthritis		
Appropriate management plan & follow-up Lifestyle advice: dietary modification; alcohol reduction; increased fluid intake NSAID +/- protein pump inhibitor until 48 hours after symptoms resolve Can consider colchicine as well Offers a review appointment to see how they are managing and to discuss long-term prophylaxis and cardiovascular risk reduction Provision of written information		
Acknowledges & addresses patient's ideas, concerns and expectations		
Gives patient opportunity to ask questions		
Examiner's Global Mark	/5	
Actor / Helper's Global Mark	/5	
Total Station Mark	/30	

Learning Points

- With any presentation it is important, while taking the history and examining a patient, to have at the forefront of your mind what are the most important differential diagnoses you need to consider and exclude. In this case you should therefore be looking to explicitly exclude red flag symptoms for septic arthritis.

- This station has a focus on clinical reasoning. It is therefore essential to know the various risk factors and precipitating factors for gout (which is largely a clinical diagnosis) and other differentials in order to make your case in support of your diagnosis.

- Patients with gout are likely to have recurrences, it is therefore important to follow them up to ensure you have conducted a medication review and discuss long term prophylaxis of allopurinol.

Chapter 8: Paediatrics

Case 1: Fever and Sore throat

Candidate's Instructions

You are the foundation year doctor working in General Practice and have been asked to see Molly who has attended the GP with her 5 year old daughter, Elizabeth, who has been brought in with a temperature, sore throat and cough. Please take a full history.

After 6 minutes the examiner will stop you and ask you to summarise back your findings, suggest your differential diagnoses and your initial management plan.

Examiner's Instructions

Molly has brought in her 5 year old daughter, Elizabeth to the GP surgery as she has a temperature, sore throat and cough.

The candidate, is acting as the foundation year doctor Doctor, and has been asked to take a history from the patient.

After 6 minutes please stop the candidate and ask them to present the case with their primary differential diagnoses. Following this ask them what their next steps regarding investigations and management will be.

If they ask, give them the examination findings below:
Examination findings:
Elizabeth is very pale and looks lethargic. She seems like she is in pain on any movement. She is currently febrile at 38.2, and has a mild tachycardia, but the rest of her observations are normal. She has bruises over her legs and arms. There is evidence of conjunctival pallor. She has widespread lymphadenopathy and hepatosplenomegaly. The rest of the clinical examination is normal including ears, nose and throat.

If they ask for the red book:
She has dropped one centile in weight since her last weigh approximately 1 year ago.

Questions to ask if there is time
What are the poor prognostic factors in Acute Lymphoblastic Leukaemia?
What are the 4 stages of treatment in ALL?

Actor's Instructions

You, Molly, have brought in your 5 year old daughter, Elizabeth, to the GP as she has a temperature, sore throat and cough.

ONLY OFFER INFORMATION IF SPECIFICALLY ASKED

Elizabeth has developed a fever over the last three days, which has been coming down with paracetamol, but yesterday she started complaining of a sore throat and is now not eating. She has had a bit of a dry cough associated with this as well. No earache, or coryzal symptoms, no vomiting or diarrhoea and her water works are normal.

This is the 4th episode of fever and sore throat she has had in the last 6 weeks. She gets better after a course of antibiotics and then just seems to get the symptoms back after the antibiotics stop. She has not needed hospital attendance yet.

She is also losing weight because she has lost her appetite especially when she has this sore throat. She is not sleeping well and seems draining of energy and not herself. She has complained of difficulty swallowing but I assumed that was due to a sore throat.

You went abroad last year to Disney World, Florida but have not been anywhere since. The strangest thing is that no one else at home seems to be catching her cold or sore throat.

She was born at 40 weeks gestation by normal vaginal delivery and there were no complications during the pregnancy or the delivery. She has never spent any time in hospital and apart from these recurrent coughs and colds has been well. She is not on any medications, has no allergies and is up to date with her immunisations. She has been developing well and met all her milestones so far.

There is a family history of eczema and asthma which your husband has. You all live together and Elizabeth has a younger brother aged 2, who is very well.

If asked about your ideas, concerns and expectations please offer the information below

You are worried that she keeps getting temperatures and getting sent home from school. You are wondering if she has a condition that is making her prone to infections or if she would benefit from her tonsils being removed. She also does not seem like the same girl, she is always tired and not as cheerful as she used to be.

Mark scheme: Fever and sore throat

Task:	Achieved	Not Achieved
Introduces himself / herself		
Confirms patient details and purpose of consultation		
Establishes the main presenting complaint		
History of presenting complaint - how many days this illness has occurred for, symptoms of infection including cough, coryza, ear ache, fevers, vomiting or diarrhoea, any urinary symptoms?		
Asks about history of other infections, what medications were needed, any hospital admissions.		
Asks about difficulty feeding or swallowing? Difficulty with breathing?		
Asks about red flags e.g. fevers, lethargy, appetite changes, night sweats		
Any unwell contacts or travel abroad?		
Asks about birth history, pregnancy history, diet & feeding		
Asks about past medical history, medication and allergies		
Asks about family history & social history		
Asks about developmental history & immunisations		
Plans to examine or asks for examination findings		
Ask for red book specifically for weight and height centiles		
Summarises findings concisely		

Able to provide appropriate differential diagnoses Normal childhood viral or bacterial infection Bone marrow disorder - leukaemia Immune deficiency condition Psychosocial - Neglect/abuse		
Suggests appropriate investigations Plot height and weight today Blood tests - FBC - identify pancytopaenia or very high WCC. Blood film, coagulation studies and U&E/LFTs - as some chemotherapy can cause deranged renal and liver function. Throat swab		
Appropriate management plan & follow-up Refer to paediatric team under 2week wait if high index of suspicion for further investigations which may include chest xray, bone marrow aspirate, lumbar puncture. Follow up with GP for psychosocial and emotional support. Multidisciplinary team involvement - social worker, psychologist, nurse specialist.		
Acknowledges & addresses patient's ideas, concerns and expectations		
Gives patient opportunity to ask questions		
Examiner's Global Mark	/5	
Actor / Helper's Global Mark	/5	
Total Station Mark	/30	

Learning Points

- Acute Leukaemia can present with very non specific symptoms that could be mistaken for an everyday fever or cold. Always consider and ask for red flag symptoms.

- When referring children to paediatric services and conducting investigations it is important to explain to parents what you want to rule out and ensure you discuss your concerns. A definitive diagnosis is not required but GPs should share their differential diagnosis with both the family and the in patient service.

- There is a good prognosis for ALL - 95% cure rate. However there are poor prognostic factors which include:

a. Total white cell count >50 X 109/L at presentation
b. Male sex
c. Philadelphia Chromosomes
d. Slow response to treatment
e. Age <1 or >10 years old
f. Afro-caribbean population

Case 2: Developmental Delay

Candidate's Instructions:

You are the foundation year doctor working in General Practice and have been asked to see Anusha who has brought in her 18month old son Tariq, because she is concerned he hasn't started walking yet. Please take a full history.

After 6 minutes the examiner will stop you and ask you to summarise back your findings, suggest your differential diagnoses and your initial management plan.

Examiner's Instructions:

Anusha has brought in her 18month old son, Tariq, because she is concerned he hasn't started walking yet.

The candidate is acting as the foundation year doctor, and has been asked to take a history from the patient.

After 6 minutes please stop the candidate and ask them to present the case with their primary differential diagnoses. Following this ask them what their next steps regarding investigations and management will be.

If they ask, give them the examination findings below:
Examination findings:
During your chat with mum, Tariq has not moved around the room at all, he is sitting up but is supporting himself with his right hand. Mum gives him a biscuit and he takes it in his right hand but then falls and cannot continue to sit upright. He has no dysmorphic features.
You conduct a neurological examination. Upper limb examination found that the left side had increased tone. Lower limb examination reveals slightly increased tone on the left, but also an upgoing plantar reflex.

If they ask for the red book:
Height and weight have remained on the 25th centile.

Questions to ask if there is time
What are the different types of cerebral palsy?

Actor's Instructions:

You are Anusha mother of 18month old Tariq, you have brought him to the GP as you are concerned that he has not started to walk yet.

ONLY OFFER INFORMATION IF SPECIFICALLY ASKED
You have been trying to encourage him to crawl by putting him on his front, or helping him stand, but he does not walk. You remember that your daughter started bottom shuffling and then started walking ages 17 months, so you were waiting for him to follow the same pattern but this did not happen. He has not bottom shuffled, he has not commando crawled, and he does not cruise around the furniture.

He has never been able to sit without support he always leans on his right arm. He rolled at about 4months.

He has always followed things around the room, he does not move things from one hand to the other, he prefers to use his right hand with which he has a pincer grip. He finds it difficult to drink from a cup.

He startles to loud noises and will turn when he hears my voice, he recognises when you say no, but will not follow one step commands easily.

He was smiling early on and enjoys playing peek a boo, with people he does not know he gets shy.

He was born at 34weeks gestation, due to placental abruption and required some time in the neonatal intensive care unit. He had difficulty breathing initially so was on a ventilator. He was treated for possible infection and also was jaundiced and needed light therapy. You cannot remember very much else. Since then he has generally been very well, never requiring hospital admission. He is currently on solid foods, and has a good appetite.

He is currently not on any medications, has no allergies and is up to date with all of his immunisations. There is no relevant family history. He lives with you, dad and 2 sisters ages 10 and 6. They are both well and thriving.

If asked about your ideas, concerns and expectations please offer the information below

You are worried as your two other children were walking by 15-17 months and using both hands, however she is worried there might be something more serious going on. He also has not started speaking yet.

Mark Scheme: Developmental Delay

Task:	Achieved	Not Achieved
Introduces himself / herself		
Confirms patient details and purpose of consultation		
Establishes main presenting complaint		
Asks about whether he bottom shuffles, commando crawls or cruises around furniture		
Developmental history: Gross Motor Skills when did he sit without support when did he roll		
Developmental history: Fine Motor & Vision Skills when did he fix and follow objects is he transferring from hand to hand does he have a pincer grip		
Developmental history: Language and Hearing recognizes voices and babbles turns to loud noises understands no obeys one step commands.		
Developmental history: Social and emotional when did he smile does he engage in social play is he now anxious with strangers can he use a cup to drink.		
Asks about birth history, pregnancy history, diet & feeding		
Asks about past medical history, medication and allergies		

Asks about family history & social history		
Asks about developmental history & immunisations		
Plans to examine or asks for examination findings		
Ask for red book specifically for weight and height centiles		
Summarises findings concisely		
Able to provide appropriate differential diagnoses Constitutional delay Global developmental delay - Cerebral Palsy Neuromuscular - muscular dystrophy Psychosocial - Neglect / Abuse		
Suggests appropriate investigations Plot height and weight today Blood tests - FBC, U&E, LFTs, TFTs - useful to have a baseline set of bloods. Special bloods - Creatinine Kinase Imaging - MRI brain		
Appropriate management plan & follow-up Multidisciplinary team approach - community paediatrician (developmental assessment), physiotherapist, neurologist, speech and language therapists, visual and hearing assessments Liaison with social services for health visitor/social workers checks.		
Acknowledges & addresses patient's ideas, concerns and expectations		
Gives patient opportunity to ask questions		
Examiner's Global Mark	/5	

Actor / Helper's Global Mark	/5	
Total Station Mark	/30	

Learning Points

- Constitutional delay is a normal variant, the average age of walking is 12-15 months. After 15 months investigations may need to be carried out. However the majority of children will be walking by age 18 months. Children who bottom shuffle or commando crawl, will be late to start walking.

- This mum is experienced as she has 3 other children at home, so she will know when something is not normal. Listen to parents, they know their child best. When parents worry you should take their concerns seriously too.

- Red flags for development include
  - Not smiling by 6 weeks
  - Unable to roll over by 6 months
  - Not sitting without support by 9 months
  - Not walking by 18 months
  - Hand preference

Case 3: Faltering growth

Candidate's Instructions:

You are the foundation year doctor working in General Practice and have been asked to see Paige who has come to see you because her 2 year old daughter, Anna is not gaining weight. Please take a full history.

After 6 minutes the examiner will stop you and ask you to summarise back your findings, suggest your differential diagnoses and your initial management plan.

Examiner's Instructions:

Paige has brought in her 2 year old daughter, Anna to the GP surgery as she is concerned about her not gaining weight.

The candidate, is acting as the foundation year doctor, and has been asked to take a history from the patient.

After 6 minutes please stop the candidate and ask them to present the case with their primary differential diagnoses. Following this ask them what their next steps regarding investigations and management will be.

If they ask, give them the examination findings below:
Examination findings:
Anna is small for a 2 year old, who looks pale and thin. She has conjunctival pallor. The chest is clear with no chest wall deformity. Heart sounds are normal.
Her abdomen is very distended and the buttocks is wasting. The abdomen is soft, with no organomegaly or masses felt. There is a scaly rash on the back of her knees.

If they ask for the red book:
Tell them that the weight has dropped from the 25th centile to the 0.4th centile. However the height has remained on the 50th centile.

Questions to ask if there is time
What other disease are associated with coeliac disease?
How can you definitively diagnose coeliac disease?
If coeliacs is confirmed what are the treatment options?

Actor's Instructions:

You, Paige, have brought in your 2 year old daughter to the GP as you are concerned she is not gaining weight. You have noticed that she seems lighter and her clothes are getting big, especially over the last 5months.

ONLY OFFER INFORMATION IF SPECIFICALLY ASKED

She has also complained of abdominal pain which is over the whole abdomen, it comes and goes, mum has noticed that it is worse after eating. It does not seem to settle with calpol. Every evening you sit together as a family and eat dinner, and it is a calm environment and she normal eats well. She has a good balanced diet with a healthy appetite, which is why you are concerned about her lack of weight gain.

She has loose stool like diarrhoea, which is foul smelling and is difficult to flush. She opens her bowels up to 4-5 times a day. There is no mucus or blood in the stool and no associated nausea or vomiting. No fevers, lethargy, appetite changes or night sweats.

Anna was born at 37 weeks gestation by elective c-section due to previous maternal C-section. There were no complications during the delivery or during the pregnancy. Anna has met all of her developmental milestones and her immunisations are up to date.

She has no past medical history of note, although has this new rash on the back of her knees which is sometimes itchy. You have been using E45 on it, but it does not seem to help. She is not on any regular medications or allergies. You have thyroid disease, but otherwise are well. There is no other relevant family history. Anna lives at home with you and her dad and an older brother, neither of whom have similar issues.

If asked about your ideas, concerns and expectations please offer the information below

You are worried that Anna may have cancer and that's why she is getting thinner and looks so pale. You would like her to be fully investigated and also like to know if there's anything you can do in order to get her to put on weight faster and if it would be worth seeing a dietician.

Mark Scheme: Faltering growth

Task:	Achieved	Not Achieved
Introduces himself / herself		
Confirms patient details and purpose of consultation		
Established the main presenting complaint & time period over which weight loss has occurred		
Asks about diet and feeding in detail - breast/bottle feeding, age of weaning, current diet, any changes to diet.		
Asks about meal times - does everyone have dinner together at the dining table, are their distractions, what happens if she does not eat?		
Asks about bowel habit - frequency, colour, consistency, smell, presence of blood/mucus		
Associated abdominal pain and history of the pain - timings of pain, nature of pain, associated symptoms e.g. nausea and vomiting, worsening symptoms with particular food.		
Asks about red flags e.g. fevers, lethargy, appetite changes, night sweats		
Asks about birth history, pregnancy history, diet & feeding		
Asks about past medical history - eczema, recurrent infections and asks about medication and allergies		
Asks about family history & social history		
Asks about developmental history & immunisations		
Plans to examine or asks for examination findings		

Ask for red book specifically for weight and height centiles		
Summarises findings concisely		
Able to provide appropriate differential diagnoses Poor feeding - behavioural Difficulty with feeding - cleft palate, neurodevelopmental delay Malabsorption - cystic fibrosis, coeliac Increased nutrient requirement - chronic illness - cardiac, respiratory, thyroid or malignancy Psychosocial - neglect		
Suggests appropriate investigations Plot height and weight today Blood tests - FBC for anaemia, U&Es for renal disease, TFTs for thyroid disease Special bloods - Coeliac antibodies Stool culture Imaging - Endoscopy and Colonoscopy may be required.		
Appropriate management plan & follow-up Keep a food diary Follow up with blood test results in 2 weeks A referral to paediatrician may be required Encourage intake of high energy foods Improve meal habits - everyone eat together, discourage force feeding.		
Acknowledges & addresses patient's ideas, concerns and expectations		
Gives patient opportunity to ask questions		
Examiner's Global Mark	/5	
Actor / Helper's Global Mark	/5	
Total Station Mark	/30	

Learning Points

- Faltering growth, previously called failure to thrive, is defined as a drop in weight by 2 centiles on a standardised growth chart. Commonest cause is due to poor intake of food that has nutritional value, which can be expected when healthier and fresher foods tend to be more expensive in the local supermarkets.

- Although in this case the history and examination point toward coeliacs, it has not yet been confirmed, therefore as a GP you have to follow up your patients, to review the problem and also to explain the results after carrying investigations. In addition you can refer to dietician and health visitors to give advice about dietary supplements and monitor the weight, respectively.

- Gold standard for investigation of coeliacs disease is a jejunal biopsy which will show villous atrophy and crypt hypertrophy. The best way to manage this condition is with a gluten free diet.

Case 4: Vaccinations

Candidate's Instructions

Claire has come to your clinic today on behalf of her daughter who is due to have a vaccination very soon. Please take a full history and then address mums ideas, concerns and expectations.

Examiner's Instructions

Claire has come to see the GP for advice and more information about the MMR vaccination. The candidate has been asked to have a conversation with the Mum which will be broken down into the following:
- History and presentation
- Discussion with mum with focus on addressing ideas, concerns and expectations

This is mostly a communication station and therefore as an examiner you can just prompt the candidate to move on to the discussion with mum.

Questions *(to be asked if there is time)*
As doctors are we allowed to act in the best interest of the child and vaccinate them? In what situations would we be allowed to act in best interest?
Can you suggest any ways in which we can prevent parents falsely interpreting information on the internet?

Actor's Instructions:

During the consultation you can either be nice or disagree with the doctor during the discussion - this station is to test their ability to communicate effectively.

You have come to the GP surgery without your daughter Amy, as you wanted to have a discussion with the doctor about the MMR vaccination.

The candidate will initially ask a number of questions about Amy to get an idea about her health.

Only offer the following information if specifically asked.

Amy is currently 1years old. She was born at 38weeks, normal delivery, no complications during pregnancy. She is currently growing well and putting on weight, she has been weaned off formula milk and eating solids.

She is meeting all her developmental milestones.
- Gross Motor: crawling, walked around holding furniture
- Fine motor: Pincer grip
- Hearing: responds to name, few words like mama, book
- Social: drinks from a cup

She has no other medical problems currently and is not on any regular medications. She did stay in hospital once due to bronchiolitis aged 6m, but she recovered well and has not been admitted since.
You have a sister who is on the autistic spectrum and some of your anxiety stems from here.
You are married and live with your husband, both of you are working and currently live in a 3bedroom house.

If asked about your ideas, concerns and expectations please offer the information below

This is your first baby and you are hoping to get some information about the MMR as everything is very controversial on the internet. She is up to date with all the other vaccines. You are worried because your sister has autism and you are unsure if that would have been related to the MMR and if that puts Amy at a higher risk of developing autism.

If the candidate tries to convince you to have the MMR, try to resist. Say that you have read an article recently on the internet, which confirmed an association between the MMR and autism, so she does not understand why we still give it.

If candidate mentions that that article was discredited, then what are the risks and benefits of the vaccine.
Please act like you have taken the information in, when the candidate explain the complications of measles, please act shocked and horrified.

You can decide if the candidate has done enough to convince you or not by the end of the consultation.

Mark Scheme: Vaccinations

Task:	Achieved	Not Achieved
Introduces himself / herself		
Confirms patient details and purpose of consultation		
Asks about birth history, pregnancy history, diet & feeding		
Asks about past medical history, medication and allergies		
Asks about family history & social history		
Asks about developmental history & immunisations		
Summarises findings concisely		
Explains the MMR vaccine and the controversy.		
Explains the discredited study		
Explains the risks and benefits of the vaccine.		
Informed mum of the new outbreak of measles this year		
Informed parents of risks and complications of measles: Corneal ulceration, Pneumonia, Suppurative otitis media, Gastroenteritis, Febrile convulsions, Encephalomyelitis (rare) and subacute sclerosing panencephalitis (very rare)		
If unsuccessful in convincing mum, gives safety net advice about concerning symptoms indicative of		

measles: typical rash, fever, conjunctivitis, koplik spots.		
Listens empathically		
Picks up on verbal cues regarding family history and asks questions regarding this		
Uses open questions throughout consultation		
Uses appropriate body language		
Avoids using medical jargon		
Acknowledges & addresses patient's ideas, concerns and expectations		
Gives patient opportunity to ask questions		
Examiner's Global Mark	/5	
Actor / Helper's Global Mark	/5	
Total Station Mark	/30	

Learning Points

- It is important to know with parents you may not always win over and convince parents of treatment. You can only ensure you have given them the appropriate information, risks and benefits. If they do not take your advice, do not give up, but ensure you safety net and make them aware of the complications. (note for more serious conditions/acute management, refusal of treatment can be taken to court or decisions made in best interest of the child)

- Measles is on the rise again, which could be due to lack of herd immunity. Therefore it is important to encourage vaccination.

- As doctors the internet is our friend, but also our biggest enemy, as the general public can now access a lot of information which may not always be interpreted correctly and therefore can make our ability to reassure and give them advice obsolete. Always point patients and parents to websites and resources which are approved or that you know provide accurate information.

Case 5: Behavioural Problems

Candidate's Instructions

You are the foundation year doctor working in General Practice and have been asked to see a stressed mum, Joy has brought her 5year old son, Thomas, as he is very active and disruptive. His behaviour is wearing her out and she is physically exhausted. Please take a full history.

After 6 minutes the examiner will stop you and ask you to summarise back your findings, suggest your differential diagnoses and your initial management plan.

Examiner's Instruction

Joy has brought in her 5year old son, Thomas to the GP surgery as she is concerned about his behaviour.

The candidate, is acting as the foundation year doctor, and has been asked to take a history from the patient.
After 6 minutes please stop the candidate and ask them to present the case with their primary differential diagnoses. Following this ask them what their next steps regarding investigations and management will be.

Examination findings: Thomas is running around the waiting room, and mum is struggling to get him to listen to her and come into the consultation room. He is very curious in the consultation room, trying to open drawers, and climb onto furniture. He interacts well with mum, but doesn't hold eye contact for very long and seems easily distractible.

Questions to ask if there is time
What is ADHD?
How do you manage a patient with ADHD?
Is there any specific medication that can be given?

Actor's Instructions

You are Joy, you have brought in your 5year old son, Thomas, as he is very active and disruptive. His behaviour is wearing you out and you are physically exhausted.

ONLY OFFER INFORMATION IF SPECIFICALLY ASKED

Over the last year Thomas has become more hyperactive, and therefore is difficult to control. He struggles to focus on one activity and is easily distractible. This has been getting worse over the last year. He also won't go to bed until midnight and sometimes later.

He behaves exactly the same at school and home. Therefore you are struggling with the teachers and school, as you have to leave work to pick him up as he upsets other children and disrupts the class.

If asked for an example of disruptive behaviour
He will sometimes in the middle of a class, get up and go for a walk and start conversations with other children who are trying to do the work given to them. He will run around the class and not listen to the teachers.

You are not concerned about his hearing or speech, he is very articulate. You are not concerned about his interactions with people, apart from sometimes he can be quite aggressive. There are no psychological stressors that could be causing any difficult behaviour, his dad left but he was very young and does not remember him. He is not being bullied at school as far as you are aware.

Thomas was born at term, no complications during the pregnancy. He was on antibiotics for the first few days of birth as you had an infection and your waters broke early. However he was discharged and he now has no other medical problems. His diet is normal, you encourage fruit and some vegetables, but he tends to eat anything.

He is not on any medications, has no allergies and his immunisations are up to date.

His cousin has ADHD and you feel like his behaviour is similar to what his mum has described. You are also a single mum with 2 children, and one child is revising for GCSEs and finding it difficult due to Thomas' behaviour.

If asked about your ideas, concerns and expectations please offer the information below

You are very concerned as Thomas is not sleeping and falling behind in school as he does not pay attention. You have come to the end of your tether and don't know what to do anymore. You are hoping there is a medication you can get to calm him down.

If you are asked about your health, wellbeing & support
You are exhausted and tired, and aren't eating very well and have lost a lot of weight. You have attributed this to stress. Your mum lives nearby but is also getting old and unable to give you as much help as before.

Mark Scheme: Behavioural Problem

Task:	Achieved	Not Achieved
Introduces himself / herself		
Confirms patient details and purpose of consultation		
Established the main presenting complaint and elicits what mum means by 'more active and hyper' & 'disruptive' Asks for examples.		
History of presenting complaint - establishes how long it has occurred for, is it getting worse, is it affecting sleep.		
Asks about school - is there variation in behaviour at school vs. home, has the school mentioned anything		
Asks about hearing or speech impairment		
Asks about his interaction and social skills with peers and family		
Ask about any psychological stressors i.e difficulty making friends, bullying, problems at home - bereavement, parental separation.		
Asks about birth history, pregnancy history, diet & feeding		
Asks about past medical history, medication and allergies		
Asks about family history & social history		
Asks about developmental history & immunisations		
Plans to examine or asks for examination findings		

Ask for red book specifically for weight and height centiles		
Summarises findings concisely		
Able to provide appropriate differential diagnoses ADHD Abuse/neglect Hearing Impairment Autism Spectrum Disorder Other Learning difficulties Bullying Normal Child - related to mums expectations		
Appropriate management & follow-up Written advice & support groups Extra support - GP to contact school and social services with consent Community paediatric referral for behavioural assessment Follow up with GP for both mum and Thomas		
Acknowledges & addresses patient's ideas, concerns and expectations		
Gives patient opportunity to ask questions		
Asks about mums support at home and addresses mums welfare. Possibly suggesting mum to come back for follow up.		
Examiner's Global Mark	/5	
Actor / Helper's Global Mark	/5	
Total Station Mark	/30	

Learning Points

- Behavioural problems can lead to a number of long term problems, including difficulty with education, inability to develop appropriate social skills and exhaustion especially if affecting sleep. However it is important to consider abuse with behavioural issues.

- Remember that with children, a parent's welfare is also important and if a mum is exhausted and not able to look after herself, she will not be able to effectively look after her child. Always check social support at home - family or friends or paid care. A social care referral may be needed to support all members of the family including the parents and siblings as well as the child concerned.

- Children should be referred to community paediatricians to do assessments, but do not forget to consider hearing or speech impairment as causes of behavioural problems and thus investigate appropriately.

Chapter 9: Obstetrics

Case 1: Antepartum Haemorrhage

Candidate's Instructions

You are the foundation year doctor working in General Practice and have been asked to see a Tania a 36 week pregnant lady, aged 29 who has presented to the GP surgery complaining of PV bleeding. Please take a full history.

After 6 minutes the examiner will stop you and ask you to summarise back your findings, suggest your differential diagnoses and your initial management plan.

Examiner's Instructions

Tania, a 36 week pregnant lady, aged 29, has presented to the GP surgery complaining of PV bleeding.

The candidate, is acting as the foundation year doctor, and has been asked to take a history from the patient.

Please note as the patient gives a history of a patient with acute bleeding, the candidate may stop and say that they would manage the patient using the Airway, breathing, circulation assessment. Just guide them to continue the history at this point.

After 6 minutes please stop the candidate at whatever stage they are and ask them to present the case with their primary differential diagnoses. Following this ask them what their next steps regarding investigations and management will be. This should take up the remaining 4 minutes of the station.

If they ask, give them the examination findings below:
Examination findings:
Mrs Totes is comfortable at rest. Her observations are currently stable.
A: Airway patent.
B: Chest clear, equal air entry bilaterally. Respiratory Rate 17 and saturations 100% on air.
C: Heart rate 87, regular and blood pressure stable at 120/86. You do not have an ECG machine.
D: GCS 15/15, Blood glucose 5.6, normal neurology. Temperature 37degrees.
E: Abdomen soft and non tender, no other signs of acute illness. No active bleeding currently.
Questions to ask if there is time:
Is there any specific diagnosis you would consider with multiple miscarriages that run in the family?

Actor's Instructions

You are Tania, a 36 week pregnant lady, aged 29, who has presented to the GP surgery complaining of PV bleeding.

ONLY OFFER INFORMATION IF SPECIFICALLY ASKED

This is your second pregnancy, and your last pregnancy unfortunately was stillborn at 30 weeks last year.

You have attended the GP as you have noticed some PV bleeding over the last week on wiping after passing urine. You do not have any urinary symptoms and you last opened your bowels this morning. Your bowel movements are normal. You do not have any abdominal pain, and you have passed fresh blood clots. No abnormal discharge recently. The bleeding has increased in intensity and frequency over the last week. This is painless bleeding. It is not associated with sex.

All blood tests have been normal throughout the pregnancy. You are Rhesus negative. Your last scan last week showed that the placenta was low and you are due another scan tomorrow as a follow up. Otherwise the scans have been normal.

You LMP (last menstrual period) was 36 weeks ago, your cycle length is normally 28 days, and is regular. Your estimated delivery date is in 2 weeks. You've not had any complications in pregnancy. You have had a few symptoms of pregnancy such as passing urine frequently and some breast tenderness.

You have had normal smear tests and no sexually transmitted infections. You have no other relevant medical history. You have no drug allergies, no regular medications. Your mother had 3 miscarriages

You are an ex-smoker, you normally drink socially, before you were pregnant. You live with you very supportive husband. You are not subject to any domestic violence at home and have never been abused.

If asked about your ideas, concerns and expectations please offer the information below

You are very anxious, given the miscarriage last year and you have looked up on the internet what PV bleeding could mean, and think that you are having another miscarriage. You feel this is what happened last time and become extremely apprehensive and tearful.

Mark scheme: Antepartum haemorrhage

Task:	Achieved	Not Achieved
Introduces himself / herself		
Confirms patient details and purpose of consultation		
Established the main presenting complaint		
Asks about bleeding - post coital bleeding, abdominal pain, pain during intercourse, abnormal discharge		
Asks about scans and blood tests during current pregnancy, including rhesus status		
Any symptoms of pregnancy - urinary, swollen legs, breast tenderness.		
Asks about past pregnancy/obstetric history		
Asks about past gynaecological history including smears and STIs		
Asks about past medical history, medications and allergies		
Asks about family history & social history including alcohol, smoking & housing		
Important to address domestic violence and abuse at home for vulnerable pregnant women at all antenatal appointments.		
Plans to examine or asks for examination findings - may ask to stabilise patient first before continuing with history.		
Candidate must not offer to do a vaginal examination as placenta praevia is suspected and can make bleeding worse		

Appreciates this may be an emergency and is able to convey this to the patient in a calm manner		
Summarises findings concisely		
Able to provide appropriate differential diagnoses Placental abruption		
Suggests appropriate investigations Routine bloods - FBC - assess blood loss, Group & Save, Clotting US Scan		
Appropriate management plan & follow-up Referral to obstetric team Review of patient following discharge from hospital (after 1week)		
Acknowledges & addresses patient's ideas, concerns and expectations		
Gives patient opportunity to ask questions		
Examiner's Global Mark	/5	
Actor / Helper's Global Mark	/5	
Total Station Mark	/30	

Learning Points

- Remember the basic structure of an obstetric history, but also do not forget to take a gynaecological history as certain factors may help in determining problems during pregnancy.

- A miscarriage (or abortion) is the loss of the fetus before 23 weeks gestation. From there onwards it would be classified as a stillbirth. In the UK 1 in 200 births ends in a stillbirth with 50% of the causes due to placental issues.

- To approach this situation calmly, realisation that it may cause the patient to worry that may worsen their symptoms. To ensure support is present and that she is accompanied to hospital. Always important to be honest regarding your thoughts on differentials.

Case 2: Proteinuria

Candidate's Instructions:

You are the foundation year doctor working in General Practice and have been asked to see a 39 week pregnant lady, Misha, aged 39 who has presented to the GP surgery for a routine antenatal appointment. Please take a focused history and perform a routine antenatal examination.

After 6 minutes the examiner will stop you and ask you to summarise back your findings, suggest your differential diagnoses and your initial management plan.

Examiner's Instructions:

A 39 week pregnant lady, Misha, aged 39 has presented to the GP surgery for a routine antenatal appointment.

The candidate, is acting as the foundation year doctor, and has been asked to take a history from the patient.

Examination findings:

Cephalic presentation
- symphysis-fundal height (SFH)- normal (39cm)
- Patient has bilateral ankle oedema
- Fetal HR normal (150bpm)
- BP High (165/110)
- Urine dip: Protein +++

All other systemic examinations are normal

After 6 minutes ask them to present the case with their primary differential diagnoses. Following this ask them what their next steps regarding investigations and management will be.

Questions to ask if there is time:
What are the risks to baby if you have pre-eclampsia?

Actor's Instructions

39 week pregnant lady, Misha, aged 39 has presented to the GP surgery for a routine antenatal appointment.

ONLY OFFER INFORMATION IF SPECIFICALLY ASKED
This is an IVF pregnancy. You have come in for a routine visit.
You have not had any headaches or visual disturbances recently. Although you have noticed your ankles swell up more so than normal since getting pregnant.
All blood tests have been normal throughout the pregnancy. You are Rhesus positive. Your scans have been normal.
You LMP (last menstrual period) was 39 weeks ago, your cycle length is normally 28 days, and is regular. You've not had any complications in pregnancy so far.
You had a termination of pregnancy when you were aged 21.
You had one abnormal smear when first tested, HPV negative and you have never had a sexually transmitted infection.

You have no other relevant medical history.
You have no drug allergies, no regular medications.
Your whole family suffer from high blood pressure, but you have never had it.
You live at home with your partner. You are a non smoker and non drinker.
You are not subject to any domestic violence at home and have never been abused.
If asked about your ideas, concerns and expectations please offer the information below
You remember at the last appointment they mentioned possible pre-eclampsia but you do not know what it means and ask the doctor to explain it to you. You become very anxious especially as it has taken you a long time to fall pregnant and this is an IVF pregnancy.

Mark scheme: Proteinuria

Task:	Achieved	Not Achieved
Introduces himself / herself		
Confirms patient details and purpose of consultation		
Established the main presenting complaint		
Asks about scans and blood tests during current pregnancy, including rhesus status		
Any symptoms of pregnancy - urinary, swollen legs		
Asks about past pregnancy/obstetric history		
Asks about past gynaecological history including smears and STIs		
Asks about past medical history		
Asks about medications and allergies		
Asks about family history & social history including alcohol, smoking & housing		
Important to address domestic violence and abuse at home for vulnerable pregnant women at all antenatal appointments.		
Acknowledges & addresses patient's ideas, concerns and expectations		
Gives patient opportunity to ask questions		
Explains what pre-eclampsia is		
Explains that the blood pressure and urine dip indicate pre-eclampsia		

Plans to examine or asks for examination findings		
Summarises findings concisely		
Able to provide appropriate differential diagnoses Likely pre-eclampsia		
Suggests appropriate investigations Blood tests to assess kidney function, electrolytes, full blood count, transaminases and bilirubin		
Appropriate management plan & follow-up Labetalol to reduce BP Ultimately patient has to give birth to resolve pre-eclampsia Warrants referral to an obstetrician for review of BP regularly Offers a review appointment to see how they are managing		
Examiner's Global Mark	/5	
Actor / Helper's Global Mark	/5	
Total Station Mark	/30	

Learning Points

- Pre-eclampsia is a raised blood pressure, with proteinuria, with or without sudden swelling of face/hands/feet, after gestation of 20 weeks.

- Labetalol is first line in managing raised BP in pregnancy.

- This can lead to an obstetric emergency and patient must be referred to an obstetrician as soon as possible.

Case 3: Antenatal check

Candidate's Instructions

You are the foundation year doctor working in General Practice and have been asked to see a 30 week pregnant lady, Debbie, aged 29, who has presented to the GP surgery for a routine antenatal appointment. Please take a focused history and perform a routine antenatal examination.

After 6 minutes the examiner will stop you and ask you to summarise back your findings, suggest your differential diagnoses and your initial management plan

Examiner's Instructions

A 30 week pregnant lady, Tina, aged 29, has presented to the GP surgery for a routine antenatal appointment.

The candidate, is acting as the foundation year doctor, and has been asked to take a history from the patient.

Examination findings:
On examination:
- Cephalic presentation
- symphysis-fundal height (SFH)- normal (30cm)
- Fetal HR normal (150bpm)
- BP normal (125/85)
- Urine dip normal

All other systemic examinations are normal.

Blood test results: 2 hour plasma glucose level: 9.1 mmol/litre

Following this prompt them to discuss their plan with the patient for 2 minutes, followed by a discussion with the examiner.

Discussion with the examiner involves asking the following questions:
How do you manage gestational diabetes?
What are the complications of gestational diabetes for the baby?

Actor's Instructions

You are a 30 week pregnant lady, Tina aged 29, who has presented to the GP surgery for a routine antenatal appointment.

ONLY OFFER INFORMATION IF SPECIFICALLY ASKED

This is your second pregnancy. You had gestational diabetes in your last pregnancy and therefore had an oral glucose tolerance test (OGTT) at your last visit and have come to discuss the results for this. You have also come in for a routine visit, which involves being examined and having your BP and urine checked.

You had an OGTT at booking and this result was normal. Today's results show that you have gestational diabetes again. You would like to try and control it with diet and exercise as this worked with your last pregnancy.

All blood tests have been normal throughout the pregnancy. You are Rhesus positive. Your scans have been normal.

You LMP (last menstrual period) was 30 weeks ago, your cycle length is normally 28 days, and is regular. You've not had any complications in pregnancy so far. You have had a few symptoms of pregnancy such as feet swelling and needing to go to pass urine many times.

You had Tom two years ago, this was a normal vaginal delivery with gestational diabetes. Baby was well and you went home from hospital the next day.

You have had normal smear tests and no sexually transmitted infections.

You have no other relevant medical history.

You have no drug allergies, no regular medications.

Your mother had gestational diabetes

You are a non smoker, you normally drink a glass of wine, but during pregnancy you have not. You live with your husband and your first child, Tom. You are not subject to any domestic violence at home and have never been abused.

If asked about your ideas, concerns and expectations please offer the information below
You are really worried about delivery as last time your baby was very big and you got a 3rd degree tear. You are wondering if this could happen again.

Mark Scheme: Antenatal Check

Task:	Achieved	Not Achieved
Introduces himself / herself		
Confirms patient details and purpose of consultation		
Established the main presenting complaint		
Asks about scans and blood tests during current pregnancy, including rhesus status		
Any symptoms of pregnancy - urinary, swollen legs, breast tenderness.		
Asks about past pregnancy/obstetric history		
Asks about past gynaecological history including smears and STIs		
Asks about past medical history		
Asks about medications and allergies		
Asks about family history & social history including alcohol, smoking & housing		
Important to address domestic violence and abuse at home for vulnerable pregnant women at all antenatal appointments.		
Plans to examine or asks for examination findings		
Explains to patient examination is normal as well as BP and urine		
Explains that the results show gestational diabetes		
Discusses management plan with patient and agrees for it to be controlled via diet/exercise		

Candidate must offer a review at the joint diabetes/antenatal clinic within a week		
Acknowledges & addresses patient's ideas, concerns and expectations		
Gives patient opportunity to ask questions		
How do you manage gestational diabetes? Self blood glucose monitoring Diet/ exercise Metformin Addition of insulin to diet/exercise/metformin Refer to dietician		
What are the complications of gestational diabetes for the baby? Macrosomia Birth trauma Shoulder dystocia Neonatal hypoglycaemia Perinatal death		
Examiner's Global Mark	/5	
Actor / Helper's Global Mark	/5	
Total Station Mark	/30	

Learning Points

- Diagnosis of gestational diabetes
    - A fasting plasma glucose level of 5.6 mmol/litre or above OR
    - A 2-hour plasma glucose level of 7.8 mmol/litre or above

- Importance that good blood glucose control throughout pregnancy will reduce the risk of fetal macrosomia, trauma during birth (for her and her baby), induction of labour and/or caesarean section, neonatal hypoglycaemia and perinatal death

- All patients diagnosed with gestational diabetes must be offered a review in a joint diabetes/antenatal clinic within a week

Case 4: Post Natal Check

Candidate's Instructions

You are the foundation year doctor working in General Practice and have been asked to see a 24 yr old lady Keely, who has had a baby 6 weeks ago, has presented to the GP surgery for her routine postnatal check. Please take a fully history.

After 6 minutes the examiner will stop you and ask you to summarise back your findings, suggest your differential diagnoses and your initial management plan.

Examiner's Instructions

A 24 yr old lady, Keely, who has had a baby 6 weeks ago, has presented to the GP surgery for her routine postnatal check.

The candidate, is acting as the foundation year doctor, and has been asked to take a history from the patient.

After 6 minutes please stop the candidate and ask them to present the case with their primary differential diagnoses. Following this ask them what their next steps regarding investigations and management will be.

If they ask, give them the examination findings below:
Examination findings:
Very quiet and withdrawn behaviour, not well kempt and thin. Looks tearful through the consultation. All other systemic examinations are normal.

Questions to ask if there is time:
What antidepressants are safe / harmful in a breastfeeding mother?
What is the importance of encouraging contraception for a short while after delivery?

Actor's Instructions

You are a 24 yr old lady, Keely, who has had a baby 6 weeks ago, has presented to the GP surgery for her routine postnatal check.

During the consultation you are very quiet and the candidate has to probe a lot before they can get any answers from you. You are reluctant to speak, and if you do, you give short answers. You avoid eye contact and look down throughout the consultation.

ONLY OFFER INFORMATION IF SPECIFICALLY ASKED

You had a normal delivery and very little blood loss. However since giving birth you have felt low in mood. You do not have any suicidal thoughts, nor have you thought of harming yourself or your baby. You have no past psychiatric history.

You are a single mum, and family live 2 hours away. You work as a waitress and you are concerned about financial care for your baby. Currently you are on maternity leave but you are anxious about funding. The midwife has visited you and she has given you information about getting financial support.

You don't have much contact with your family. You remember your mum mentioning having postnatal depression but not sure. You feel very lonely and isolated. None of your friends have any children and you have found it more difficult to socialize with them. You have not experienced any of the following symptoms - headache, palpitations, feeling too hot/cold, loose bowels/constipation, weakness.

You have no other relevant medical history. You have no drug allergies, no regular medications. You are a non smoker and you normally drink a glass of wine every night.

If asked about your ideas, concerns and expectations please offer the information below
You have been very tired and feel guilty as you think you are not looking after your baby properly. You feel worthless. You do not know what to do anymore and are hoping that the doctor can provide some support. You are open to getting help and support and will return for a follow up appointment if offered.

Case 3: Postnatal check

Task:	Achieved	Not Achieved
Introduces himself / herself		
Confirms patient details and purpose of consultation		
Established the main presenting complaint		
Uses open questions to start consultation		
Uses silence as a tool make patient feel she can take her time		
Enquires about mood (Edinburgh postnatal depression scale) Able to laugh/see funny side of things? Look forward with enjoyment to things? Blames herself unnecessarily? Anxious/worried for no good reason? Felt scared/panicky? Things have been getting on top of her? Difficulty sleeping? Crying? Felt sad/miserable?		
Asks sensitively about thoughts of self harm/suicide		
Systemic review- headache, palpitations, feeling too hot/cold, loose bowels/constipation, weakness		
Social history specifically support at home, financial status, nutrition for herself and baby, accommodation		
Important to address domestic violence and abuse at home for vulnerable pregnant women at all antenatal appointments.		
Asks about past medical history		
Asks about medications and allergies		

Asks about family history		
Plans to examine or asks for examination findings		
Summarises findings concisely		
Able to provide appropriate differential diagnoses Postnatal depression Postnatal blues Thyroid problems (postpartum thyroiditis)		
Suggests appropriate investigations Blood tests to review thyroid function		
Appropriate management plan & follow-up Offers a review appointment to see how they are managing. Considers starting antidepressant (safe in breastfeeding) Considers counselling at a mother and baby unit Follow up to discuss contraception methods and blood pressure review as well.		
Acknowledges & addresses patient's ideas, concerns and expectations		
Gives patient opportunity to ask questions		
Examiner's Global Mark	/5	
Actor / Helper's Global Mark	/5	
Total Station Mark	/30	

Learning Points

- Although the instructions say to do postnatal check-up, you have to be aware the station is more to recognise this lady's postnatal depression and assess the risk and severity. You can always mention at the end 'We can complete the check up on our follow up appointment'.

- To assess severity of postnatal depression you can make yourself familiar with Edinburgh postnatal depression scale (EPDS). Baby blues are very common self limiting feelings after birth but if more protracted and deep set emotions exist then true postpartum depression needs to be considered.
- Remember the safety of the baby, are you happy for this mother's care for the baby. If not, mention you will escalate to a senior. If you suspect mental health issues the involvement of social care can lend support to both the mother and baby.

Chapter 10: Gynaecology

Case 1: Sexually transmitted infections

Candidate's Instructions

You are the foundation year doctor working in General Practice and have been asked to see a 19 year old, Natalie who has presented to the GP surgery due to a personal problem. Please take a full history.

After 6 minutes the examiner will stop you and ask you to summarise back your findings, suggest your differential diagnoses and your initial management plan.

Examiner's Instructions

A 19 year old, Natalie has presented to the GP surgery due to a personal problem.

The candidate, is acting as the foundation year doctor Doctor, and has been asked to take a history from the patient. After 6 minutes please stop the candidate and ask them to present the case with their primary differential diagnoses. Following this ask them what their next steps regarding investigations and management will be.
If they ask, give them the examination findings below:

Examination findings:

Natalie is comfortable and observations are normal. On examination, there is some frothy discharge PV, which has a fish like odour. When using a speculum you find a strawberry cervix. All other systemic examinations are normal.
Questions to ask if there is time:
What is contact tracing?
What are the complications of untreated sexually transmitted diseases?

Actor's Instructions:

You are a 19 year old Natalie, who has presented to the GP surgery due to a personal problem.

ONLY OFFER INFORMATION IF SPECIFICALLY ASKED

You have come to see your GP today because you are very worried about some concerns "down below" that you are anxious and nervous about discussing. You're reluctant initially and say you want a "check-up".

Ten days ago, you returned from a holiday to Spain with your university friends. You haven't been feeling very well since coming back. On further probing you mention that you have made a mistake.

You explain that before your holiday you had recently broken up with your boyfriend of 2 years, Chris. While out in Spain you had a one night stand with a man you met at the clubs. It involved penetrative sex. You did not use protection. No other people were involved. You feel awful and embarrassed about it, especially that now Chris wants you back.

You are worried about some frothy yellow-green discharge that you've been having. The discharge smells unpleasant, almost like fish. Your area "down below" is very itchy. As a result it is very sore and red. You also get some burning when passing urine.
While with Chris, you used condoms and you also took the COCP. You have not stopped it because you have been so used to taking it.

Your periods are generally regular. They come every 23-25 days or so. You would be bleeding for 6 days each time; and it is not heavy. You have some back pain in the first day but this subsides on its own.

You had an abortion when you were 17 as a condom split and you have been careful since. You do not have any health problems and never saw a gynaecologist. You take no regular medications and have no allergies. You've had all your immunisations including the HPV vaccine. You haven't had a smear yet.

You smoke 10 a day and drink socially. You have tried cannabis once and did not like it. You have no relevant family history.

If asked about your ideas, concerns and expectations please offer the information below

You are concerned this could be an STI and want to have it treated. You're not sure if you are going to have to tell Chris.

Mark Scheme: Sexually transmitted infections

Task:	Achieved	Not Achieved
Introduces himself / herself		
Confirms patient details and purpose of consultation		
Established the main presenting complaint		
Asks about local symptoms: Discharge- colour, smell Itching Pain, dyspareunia (deep/superficial) Genital skin changes- rash, blisters, redness		
Asks about systemic symptoms: Abdominal pain, Urinary symptoms, Other rashes, Arthritis, Uveitis, Pyrexia, Weight loss		
Take a menstrual history: Last menstrual period, Regularity, Cycle length, Menorrhagia, Post coital bleeding, Intermenstrual bleeding		
Asks about previous and current contraception		
Elicit past gynae history: pregnancies, terminations, operations, STIs		
Specifically asks about smear tests		
Asks about current relationship & sexual history: - Last sexual contact - Number of partners, long term vs. casual - Consensual - Type of sex - Contraception - Age of partner - Sexual history of partner/HIV risk		
Asks about past medical history		

Asks about medications and allergies		
Asks about family history & social history including alcohol and smoking		
Plans to examine or asks for examination findings		
Summarises findings concisely		
Able to provide appropriate differential diagnoses **Trichomoniasis** Bacterial Vaginosis Gonorrhoea		
Suggests appropriate investigations Swabs inc. high vaginal swab Urine MC&S Pregnancy test		
Appropriate management plan & follow-up Antibiotics (Metronidazole) Sexual intercourse avoided for at least 1week Treat partner Offers a review appointment to see how they are managing.		
Acknowledges & addresses patient's ideas, concerns and expectations		
Gives patient opportunity to ask questions		
Examiner's Global Mark	/5	
Actor / Helper's Global Mark	/5	
Total Station Mark	/30	

Learning Points

- When asking about symptoms, ensure to enquire about discharge: colour, consistency and smell as this often leads you to the diagnosis.

- When asking about sexual history, think of the 5 P's of sexual health: Partner, Practices, Protection, Past history, Prevention of pregnancyˇ. Do not forget to discuss contact tracing (if required) when asking about the partner.

- Not all patients are comfortable discussing their sexual history. Try to overcome this with open questioning style and focusing on patient's cues. Also try reiterating confidentiality and that the questions are for all patients with sexual related complaints. Offer a chaperone if it would make the patient more comfortable.

ˇRef: US Department Of Health And Human Services Centers For Disease Control And Prevention, a guide to taking a sexual history

Case 2: Cervical Smear

Candidate's instructions

You are the foundation year doctor in the GP and have been asked to see Tessa a 28 year old woman, has been asked to come to the GP surgery to discuss the results of a recent cervical smear. The result shows mild dyskaryosis and HPV Type 16 (high risk) positive.

Take a focused history and discuss the results with the patient and then suggest an appropriate management plan and address their ideas, concerns and expectations.

Examiner Instructions

Tessa, a 28 year old woman, has been asked to come to the GP surgery to discuss the results of a recent cervical smear. The result shows mild dyskaryosis and HPV Type 16 (high risk) positive. The patient is unaware of the results.

The candidate, is acting as the foundation year doctor, and has been asked to take a brief history from the patient.

Questions to ask if there is time:
What are the stages of CIN and when does it become cancer?
What treatments can be offered at different stages?

Actor instructions

You are Tessa, a 28 year old woman, who has been asked to come to the GP surgery to discuss the results of a recent cervical smear. You were not told anything about the nature of the results and you have assumed the worst. You are very anxious and emotional about hearing the results.

ONLY OFFER INFORMATION IF SPECIFICALLY ASKED

This was your second smear. You had your first three years ago which was normal. Your mother convinced you of the importance of having the smears done but you have little understanding of the tests or the nature of the disease apart from thinking it is a test for cervical cancer.

You have had no symptoms recently. In particular you have had no vaginal discharge, no bleeding after sex, and no bleeding between periods. You have not noticed any change in your appetite or weight.

You have no known ongoing medical problems. You take no regular medication except the oral contraceptive pill which you have been taking since you were seventeen. You have no allergies.

You do not think you had a vaccine as a child to prevent cervical cancer.
Your mother had an abnormal smear result in her thirties and had a minor operation.
You are a social smoker, smoking roughly 5-10 cigarettes per week. You rarely drink alcohol. You work as a hairdresser. You live with a friend. You are currently single but sexually active. You have had around ten sexual partners in your life.

If asked about your ideas, concerns and expectations please offer the information below

You are very anxious about the results and you think the doctor is going to tell you that you have cancer.

Take a little time to process the news that the results are abnormal before being ready to continue talking.

The candidate will take some time to address your specific questions:

- You want to understand the nature of the test and what the results mean. You are happy to let the candidate explain the results as they see fit.
- If there is time, ask how you got the virus. You are concerned about what you might have done to cause these abnormal results and feel that it is your fault.

If the candidate talks at you and/or talk in a manner that you don't easily understand then appear confused. If they do not pick up on this after a minute or so then interrupt them.

If the candidate does not speak to you empathically then confront them about this – you may become angry at their lack of empathy.

Mark scheme: Cervical Smear

Task:	Achieved	Not Achieved
Introduces himself / herself		
Confirms patient details and purpose of consultation		
Asks about local symptoms: Discharge- colour, smell Itching Pain, dyspareunia (deep/superficial) Genital skin changes- rash, blisters, redness		
Specifically asks about previous smear tests		
Detailed sexual history: Last sexual contact Consensual Partner- number, gender, paid, abroad Type of sex Contraception Other partners in last 3 months HIV risk		
Asks about past medical history, medications and allergies		
Asks about family history & social history including alcohol and smoking		
Finds out what patient's understanding is thus far		
Gives a warning shot		
Gives clear information regarding the results and avoids use of jargon		
Uses silence as a tool, before continuing with consultation		

Uses appropriate body language		
Clearly explains in simple terms that mild dyskaryosis is a warning that there is a risk of developing cancer but does not mean the patient has cancer		
Clearly explains that the HPV virus causes the dyskaryosis and that it is of a type associated with higher risk of developing cancer		
Correctly identifies colposcopy as the next step and is able to briefly explain what this entails		
Acknowledges & addresses patient's ideas, concerns and expectations		
Smoking cessation with explanation (specifically that smoking can increase risk of developing cervical cancer)		
Summarises results and actions from here on and checks for understanding and questions		
Offers additional written material		
Gives patient opportunity to ask questions		
Examiner's Global Mark	/5	
Actor / Helper's Global Mark	/5	
Total Station Mark	/30	

Learning Points

- When delivering any kind of news, in this case cervical smear results, the same basic structure is helpful. This is a difficult situation, however, as smear results need some explanation. Patients often wants the results straight away, and stalling over giving them the results can anger them, but hearing the results without an understanding of their meaning can cause undue anxiety and distress. All clinicians will approach this slightly differently and it's important that you find your own style that feels and sounds natural.

- Rather than blindside the patient with the news, always remember to give a "warning shot" and then pause for a moment. Keep it simple – "I have some bad news" may sound cliché but it suffices. Find your own way of saying it.

- Pacing your delivery is vital. Give small chunks of information at a time. Pay attention to non-verbal cues – are they nodding along or do they look confused or upset? Pauses are also a chance for you to intermittently check in with them actively.

Case 3: Contraception

Candidate's Instructions

You are the foundation year doctor working in General Practice and have been asked to see a 17 year old lady, Nadia who has presented to the GP surgery and would like to discuss her options regarding contraception.

Please take a history and address the patient's ideas, concerns and expectations and then suggest her contraception options.

Examiner's Instructions

A 17 year old lady Nadia, has presented to the GP surgery and would like to discuss her options regarding contraception.

The candidate, is acting as the foundation year doctor Doctor, and has been asked to take a history from the patient.

The candidate should discuss their next steps regarding management and address patients ideas, concerns and expectations. The candidate should also I counsel the patient with regards to the risks and benefits of her chosen option.

Questions to ask if there is time:
How does the COCP pill work in terms of the hormonal impact?
What do you advise a patient to do if they miss a pill?

Actor's Instructions

You are a 17 year old lady Nadia, who has presented to the GP surgery and would like to discuss her options regarding contraception.

ONLY OFFER INFORMATION IF SPECIFICALLY ASKED

You have come to see your GP today because you have been with your current 18 year old boyfriend for 5 months and you are looking to start another method of contraception as neither of you like condoms.

Your current boyfriend is your only partner. You last had sexual contact a week ago and this was penetrative sex. You are happy in this relationship and sex is always consensual You have always used condoms. You do not know very much about your partner's previous sexual history but suspect he has had other partners.

Your periods are painful but not overly heavy. They are regular and your last period was 2 weeks ago.

You are generally fit and well. You have well controlled asthma and only use salbutamol inhaler in the winter. You have never been pregnant or needed to see the gynaecologist. You take no regular medications and have no allergies. You've had all your immunisations including the HPV vaccine. You haven't had a smear yet.

You have no relevant family history. You smoke 10 a day and drink socially.

If asked about your ideas, concerns and expectations please offer the information below

You do not know a lot about contraception as you were away when they had that lesson at school and your knowledge is from the internet. You know unprotected sex can lead to pregnancy and STIs. You know friends who are on the pill and have claimed it is so easy so you are keen to try it. However you would like to know the side effects as you are worried they will make your spots worse and make you put on weight.

Mark scheme: Contraception

Task:	Achieved	Not Achieved
Introduces himself / herself		
Confirms patient details and purpose of consultation		
Asks about current relationship & sexual history: - Last sexual contact - Number of partners, long term vs. casual - Consensual - Type of sex - Contraception - Age of partner - Sexual history of partner/HIV risk		
Take a menstrual history: Last menstrual period, Regularity, Cycle length, Menorrhagia, Post coital bleeding, Intermenstrual bleeding		
Elicit past gynae history: pregnancies, terminations, operations, STIs		
Asks about previous and current contraception		
Specifically asks about smear tests		
Asks about past medical history		
Asks about medications and allergies		
Asks about family history (VTE, breast cancer)		
Asks about social history including alcohol and smoking		
Establish patient's baseline knowledge and preferences about contraception		
Offer methods at least 3 methods of contraception COCP, POP, implant, Depo, IUCD		

Explain how the COCP works		
Explain the benefits of COCP: - Very effective contraceptive - More regular, lighter, less painful periods - Reduced risk of ovarian, endometrial, bowel cancers + risk of fibroids, ovarian cysts, benign breast cysts		
Explain the risks of COCP: - Nausea - Headache - Breast tenderness - Weight gain - Very rare risk of VTE and MI		
Checks patient's understanding of information given		
Provides written information		
Acknowledges & addresses patient's ideas, concerns and expectations		
Gives patient opportunity to ask questions		
Examiner's Global Mark	/5	
Actor / Helper's Global Mark	/5	
Total Station Mark	/30	

Learning Points

- When discussing contraception options it is important to ensure maximal compliance. Firstly consider the safety of the method from a medical perspective by taking a full medical and family history, as well as examining the patient. If there are contraindications, explain this to the patient. Also consider the acceptability of the contraceptive to the patient and how it fits into their lifestyle.

- It is important that patients on the pill take it reliably and accurately. There are a number of rules to consider. If the pill is late < 24hrs, patient can take the pill and continue as normal. If ONE pill is missed for >24hrs, take the pill when remembered (even if 2 pills at once) and continue as normal. If TWO or more pills are missed, take the last pill when remembered (even if 2 pills at once) and use barrier contraception. If at the last 7 days of the pack, continue to next pack without a break.

- When counselling women about the pill ensure to cover: major complications their symptoms and when to seek help, the benefits, smoking and cessation advice, and highlight the importance of regular review and blood pressure monitoring.

Case 4: Menorrhagia

Candidate's Instructions

You are the foundation year doctor working in General Practice and have been asked to see a A 28 year old Claire who has presented to the GP to discuss her periods as she is very concerned about them becoming heavier than usual.

After 6 minutes the examiner will stop you and ask you to summarise back your findings, suggest your differential diagnoses and your initial management plan.

Examiner's Instructions:

A 28 year old Claire, has presented to the GP to discuss her periods as she is very concerned about them becoming heavier than usual.

The candidate, is acting as the foundation year doctor, and has been asked to take a history from the patient.

After 6 minutes please stop the candidate and ask them to present the case with their primary differential diagnoses. Following this ask them what their next steps regarding investigations and management will be. T

Questions to ask if there is time:
What is the mechanism of action of tranexamic acid?

Actor's Instructions

You are A 28 year old Claire, who has presented to the GP to discuss her periods as you are concerned about them becoming heavier than usual.

ONLY OFFER INFORMATION IF SPECIFICALLY ASKED

You have come to see your GP today because you are at the end of your tether with your periods.

For the last 6 months or so your periods are becoming increasingly heavier. You are having to change your pads every hour and you have had many occasions of flooding. It has made your daily life very difficult that you have had to take time off work, as an accountant, and work from home recently because of embarrassment.

Your periods are generally regular. They come every 30-32 days or so. You would be bleeding for 8-10 days each time; and it is heavy throughout. You have extreme back pain in the first 3 days but this subsides with paracetamol on the fourth day.

You are currently in between relationships and have only just started seeing a new man but you have not had sexual intercourse yet. You are not planning to conceive at the moment. When asked about contraception, you were on the COCP and that caused you to breakout in acne and have headaches so you have stopped it. You are hoping to use condoms in your new relationship and consider alternatives later.

You were invited for smear test but never managed to arrange an appointment.

You had Chlamydia when you were 17 but that has cleared and you have been careful since. You do not have any health problems and never saw a gynaecologist.

You have no other medical problems. You take no regular medications and you are allergic to penicillin (rash). You have no relevant family history.

If asked about your ideas, concerns and expectations please offer the information below

You have googled what this could be and you are worried it could be womb or cervical cancer.

Mark Scheme: Menorrhagia

Task:	Achieved	Not Achieved
Introduces himself / herself		
Confirms patient details and purpose of consultation		
Established the main presenting complaint		
Take a menstrual history: Last menstrual period, Regularity, Cycle length, Menorrhagia, Post coital bleeding, Intermenstrual bleeding		
Asks about amount of bleeding: flooding, clots		
Asks about pain		
Ellicit impact on daily life		
Briefly asks about sexual history		
Asks about previous and current contraception		
Specifically asks about smear tests		
Ellicit past gynae history: pregnancies, terminations, operations, STIs		
Asks about past medical history specifically about bleeding tendencies or thyroid disorders		
Asks about medications and allergies		
Asks about family history & social history including alcohol and smoking		
Summarises findings concisely		
Able to provide appropriate differential diagnoses Dysfunctional uterine bleeding Fibroids Polyps		

Endometriosis IUCD Hypothyroidism		
Suggests appropriate investigations Bloods to exclude anaemia & systemic causes (clotting and TFTs) Smear test TVUS		
Appropriate management plan & follow-up If trying to conceive – tranexamic acid or NSAIDs. If not trying to conceive – Progestogen IUS or COCP Offers a review appointment to see how they are managing.		
Acknowledges & addresses patient's ideas, concerns and expectations		
Gives patient opportunity to ask questions		
Examiner's Global Mark	/5	
Actor / Helper's Global Mark	/5	
Total Station Mark	/35	

Learning Points

- To help with assessing menstrual disorders, divide them to heavy, irregular or no bleeding. Therefore assessing the timing and amount is very important.

- Good history taking is essential to identify the causes of menorrhagia, particularly as dysfunctional uterine bleeding is a diagnosis of exclusion. Exclude local and systemic causes first.

- Always consider the impact of such conditions on patients life. Can be psychologically taxing and difficult to cope with.

Case 5: Infertility

Candidate's Instructions

You are the foundation year doctor working in General Practice and have been asked to see a 27 year old lady, Sania who has presented to the GP surgery to discuss conception. Please take a full history.

After 6 minutes the examiner will stop you and ask you to summarise back your findings, suggest your differential diagnoses and your initial management plan.

Examiner's Instructions

A 27 year old lady Sania, has presented to the GP surgery to discuss conception.

The candidate, is acting as the foundation year doctor, and has been asked to take a history from the patient.

After 6 minutes please stop the candidate and ask them to present the case with their primary differential diagnoses. Following this ask them what their next steps regarding investigations and management will be.

Questions to ask if there is time:
What are the diagnostic criteria for polycystic ovary syndrome?
What are the criteria for referral to fertility services for IVF?

Actor's Instructions

You are a 27 year old lady Sania who has presented to the GP surgery to discuss conception.

ONLY OFFER INFORMATION IF SPECIFICALLY ASKED

You have come to see your GP today because you and your husband have been trying for a baby for over 10 months and you are very worried you may be infertile and never have children.

You have been married for 3 years and started having unprotected penetrative sexual intercourse 2-3 times a week for 8 months. You are not sure when it falls during your cycle but you have tried to time it with the over the counter testing strips. You have not had any problems with pain or bleeding having sex.

Your last period was 1.5 months ago. Your periods are actually irregular, you can go 2 months without one. You would be bleeding for 10 days each time; and it is quite heavy, changing pads every 3 hours or so. You have some back pain in the first day but this subsides with some paracetamol.

You had a miscarriage once when you first got married but you have not had any other pregnancies. You have never had to see a gynaecologist. You had your smear test and it was normal.

You have always struggled with acne but it seemed to be getting worse in the last year. You have been trying to shed some weight since college but have been struggling. When you asked, you do think you are hairy but you have always put it to genes and not thought much of it. You are otherwise well and do not suffer with headaches or nipple discharge. You have no medical problems and have only been taking folic acid. You have no allergies. You do not smoke or drink alcohol. Your mother has diabetes.

Your partner is a 30 year old school teacher. He does not have any other children from previous relationships. He has no medical problems and does not take any medications. He is a smoker of 15/day.

If asked about your ideas, concerns and expectations please offer the information below
You are concerned that you will never be able to have children. You are anxious but settle after reassurance.

Mark scheme: Infertility

Task:	Achieved	Not Achieved
Introduces himself / herself		
Confirms patient details and purpose of consultation		
Established the main presenting complaint		
Asks about duration of unprotected intercourse		
Asks about intercourse: type, frequency, when in cycle		
Asks about problems with intercourse: pain, bleeding		
Take a menstrual history: Last menstrual period, Regularity, Cycle length, Menorrhagia, Intermenstrual bleeding		
Elicits past gynae history: pregnancies, terminations, operations, STIs		
Asks about Polycystic ovary syndrome symptoms: Hirsutism, acne, weight gain		
Asks about hyperprolactinaemia symptoms: Nipple discharge, headaches		
Specifically asks about smear tests		
Asks about past medical history, medications and allergies		
Asks about family history & social history including alcohol and smoking		
Asks about partner: age, occupation, previous children, smoking/drugs, medications		
Summarises findings concisely		

Able to provide appropriate differential diagnoses **Polycystic ovary syndrome** Hypothyroidism Hyperprolactinaemia		
Suggests appropriate investigations Bloods (FSH, LH, prolactin, TSH, testosterone) Transvaginal ultrasound scan Fasting lipids and glucose		
Appropriate management plan & follow-up Inform them of the criteria for infertility referral, so if needed one day they are prepared includes - Diet & exercise (BMI), smoking. Medical mx: metformin, clomifen Offers a review appointment to see how they are managing.		
Acknowledges & addresses patient's ideas, concerns and expectations		
Gives patient opportunity to ask questions		
Examiner's Global Mark	/5	
Actor / Helper's Global Mark	/5	
Total Station Mark	/30	

Learning Points

- When considering conception, infertility is defined as inability to conceive following at least 12 months of unprotected intercourse. Some cases of infertility require referral to specialist services if:

    - Not conceived after 1 year in with no known cause of infertility
    - Had 6 cycles of artificial insemination and no known cause of infertility
    - Woman is aged >36 years old with a cause of infertility

- Infertility can be primary, i.e. never conceived, or secondary previously conceived. As the differentials for each are different it is important to ask about previous pregnancies or children for both partners.

- When managing PCOS, it is important to consider if the woman is trying to conceive or not. If the woman is trying to conceive the mainstay of treatment is clomifene and metformin. However if conception is not an issue, medications such as Co-cyprindriol and COCP are more important.

Case 6: Post menopausal bleeding

Candidate's Instructions

You are the foundation year doctor working in General Practice and have been asked to see a 52 year old lady Jane who has presented to the GP surgery complaining of some bleeding she has been having. Please take a full history.

After 6 minutes the examiner will stop you and ask you to summarise back your findings, suggest your differential diagnoses and your initial management plan.

Examiner's Instructions

A 52 year old lady, Jane O'Brian, has presented to the GP surgery complaining of some bleeding she has been having.
The candidate, is acting as the foundation year doctor Doctor, and has been asked to take a history from the patient.

After 6 minutes please stop the candidate and ask them to present the case with their primary differential diagnoses. Following this ask them what their next steps regarding investigations and management will be.

If they ask, give them the examination findings below:
Examination findings:
Mrs O'Brien is comfortable at rest and her observations are normal. On examination abdomen is soft non tender, no masses felt. PV examination is normal.
All other systemic examinations are normal.
Questions to ask if there is time:
What are the side effects of hormone replacement therapy?

Actor's Instructions:

You are 52 year old lady, Jane O'Brian, who has presented to the GP surgery complaining of some bleeding she has been having.

ONLY OFFER INFORMATION IF SPECIFICALLY ASKED

You have come to see your GP today because you are very worried about some concerns "down below". You have been bleeding intermittently for the last 3 weeks. You are very puzzled because you had stopped having periods a year and a half ago.
The bleeds are unpredictable. It happened once 3 weeks ago, then once again last week. You didn't think much of it initially. However this week you have been bleeding continuously for 3 days. Initially the bleeding was light, but now it is getting heavier; you need 2 pads per day. It looks like periods and there are no clots. You have been having some watery discharge in the interim. You have never had this before.

You are glad it is not painful like periods. You are sexually active and have not had any pain or bleeding relating to sexual intercourse. Nor have you felt any lumps. You have not had any pessaries or examinations recently.

Your last period was 1.5 years ago. You started periods when you were 11. Your periods were generally regular, every 25-29 days or so. You would be bleeding for 5 days each time; and it is not heavy. You have some back pain in the first day but this subsides with some paracetamol.

You had an abortion when you were 17 but you have not had any other pregnancies. You have never had to see a gynaecologist. You had your smear tests regularly and you had low grade changes once, around 6 years ago.

You have diet controlled diabetes. You take no regular medications apart from HRT and have no allergies. Your HRT is a patch that you started 1 year ago and it is continuous therapy as you did not want to have more periods.

You smoke 5-10 a day and drink socially. You have an aunt who had breast cancer.

If asked about your ideas, concerns and expectations please offer the information below

You are concerned this could be cancer because you looked on google and would like all the tests possible to find out.

Mark Scheme: Post menopausal bleeding

Task:	Achieved	Not Achieved
Introduces himself / herself		
Confirms patient details and purpose of consultation		
Established the main presenting complaint		
Asks about onset, timing of bleeding, colour and amount of bleeding: flooding, clots		
Asks about local trauma (e.g. recent pessary, cervical biopsy, etc) or external symptoms (discharge, rashes, lumps)		
Asks about systemic symptoms: Abdo pain, Urinary symptoms		
Asks about red flag symptoms - weight loss, loss of appetite, lethargy, night sweats, fevers		
Take a menstrual history: Last menstrual period, Regularity, Cycle length, Menorrhagia, Post coital bleeding, Intermenstrual bleeding		
Elicits past gynae history: pregnancies, terminations, operations, STIs		
Asks about Hormone replacement therapy: how long, continuous/cyclical, effect on bleeding		
Specifically asks about smear tests		
Asks about past medical history, medications and allergies		
Asks about family history & social history including alcohol and smoking		
Plans to examine or asks for examination findings		
Summarises findings concisely		

Able to provide appropriate differential diagnoses **Endometrial cancer** Cervical cancer/polyps Withdrawal bleed with HRT Atrophic vaginitis		
Suggests appropriate investigations Cervical smear Transvaginal ultrasound scan Hysteroscopy		
Appropriate management plan & follow-up 2 week wait referral to gynaecology Offers a review appointment to see how they are managing.		
Acknowledges & addresses patient's ideas, concerns and expectations		
Gives patient opportunity to ask questions		
Examiner's Global Mark	/5	
Actor / Helper's Global Mark	/5	
Total Station Mark	/30	

Learning Points

- Post menopausal bleeding is considered when it is 12 months after the last period. Therefore it is important to take a detailed menstrual history, first to establish menopause and PMB.

- Hormone replacement therapy (HRT) can be administered with care. Always consider the risks vs the symptomatic benefits, particularly in those over the age of 60 years. Consider cyclical preparations vs. continuous as this case may represent an oestrogen withdrawal bleed. HRT increases the risk VTE and of breast (not if oestrogen only) and endometrial (if oestrogen only) cancers. However it reduced the risk of colon cancer.

- Dealing with anxious patients is a skill that is tested in OSCE. Ensure you are patient centred and deal with the concerns appropriately. By identifying their ideas and concerns early, this will help you structure your consultation and

Chapter 11: Psychiatry

Case 1: Depression

Candidate instructions

You are the foundation year doctor working in General Practice and have been asked to see a 33 yr old woman Millie who has presented to the GP surgery complaining of difficulty sleeping. Please take a full history.

After 6 minutes the examiner will stop you and ask you to summarise back your findings, suggest your differential diagnoses and your initial management plan.

Examiner Instructions

A 33 yr old woman Millie has presented to the GP surgery complaining of difficulty sleeping.

The candidate, is acting as the foundation year doctor, and has been asked to take a history from the patient.

After 6 minutes please stop the candidate and ask them to present the case with their primary differential diagnoses. Following this ask them what their next steps regarding investigations and management will be.

Questions to ask if there is time:

What caution do you need to give if starting an antidepressant? What are the side effects?

Actor's Instructions

You are a 33 yr old woman Millie who has presented to the GP surgery complaining of difficulty sleeping.

ONLY OFFER INFORMATION IF SPECIFICALLY ASKED

For the past 6 months you have been feeling increasingly run down and lacking in energy, which you think is because you haven't been sleeping very well. You go to bed at around midnight but find it very difficult to get to sleep. You are finding that you are constantly waking up in the middle of the night and wake before your alarm goes off. During the day, you feel very tired and have problems concentrating. Last month you fell asleep in a meeting which was attended by some important clients. You are an investment banker working in the city. Your manager was also in attendance and took you aside after the meeting- you have a good working relationship with her but she warned you that if it happened again, she would have to escalate it further.

You used to be a very sociable person but haven't felt up to joining your colleagues for drinks at the end of the week, and would rather stay at home. You also used to enjoy going to the gym but this has stopped.

Your partner has an equally busy job so sometimes you don't see each other for a few days. You don't want to mention any of this to him/her as you don't want them to think you are a failure. You are not particularly close to your family and they live quite far away so you don't see them often, and your friends all seem to be busy with their own lives.

You have felt that your mood is low and sometimes you feel tearful. You have not had any thoughts of harming yourself or ending your life. You have never heard any voices or seen anything that wasn't there.

You don't smoke and you drink approximately 3 bottles of wine throughout the week. You haven't had much of an appetite and have lost a bit of weight. You are usually fit and healthy and haven't had to see your GP before. You do not take any medication. Both of your parents have high cholesterol and you think your aunt suffered from depression for which she took medication.

If asked about your ideas, concerns and expectations please offer the information below

You feel that the problems with sleeping were triggered due to an email stating the company would be restructuring and that some people may lose their jobs. You have just bought a house with your partner and have a mortgage to pay which is just about covered by your salaries.

You think it might be stress that is keeping you awake but you also think you may be depressed. You would like the GP to offer you support and direct you to services where you can talk to someone. You would also like something to help you sleep at night.

Mark Scheme: Depression

	Achieved	Not Achieved
Introduces himself / herself		
Confirms patient details and purpose of consultation		
Established the main presenting complaint		
Asks about sleeping pattern during the night		
Asks if there is anything that may have caused trouble sleeping		
Asks about impact on work life		
Asks about having problems concentrating		
Asks about impact on social life		
Asks about low mood, finding little interest or pleasure in doing things, hopelessness		
Assesses suicidal risk by asking specifically about thoughts of self harm		
Asks specifically about hearing or seeing things which aren't there		
Asks about eating and appetite		
Asks about past medical history, medications and allergies		
Asks about family history & social history including alcohol and smoking		
Summarises findings concisely		
Able to provide appropriate differential diagnoses Depression Sleep disturbance Anxiety		

Appropriate management plan & follow-up Cognitive behavioural therapy Antidepressants Offers a review appointment to see how they are managing and to assess suicidal risk.		
Offers written information and helplines in case of emergency		
Acknowledges & addresses patient's ideas, concerns and expectations		
Gives patient opportunity to ask questions		
Examiner's Global Mark	/5	
Actor / Helper's Global Mark	/5	
Total Station Mark	/30	

Learning Points

- In Primary Care, there are tools which can help to screen patients for depression. The Patient Health Questionnaire (PHQ-2) is a two question screening tool that the patient completes as a 'first-step' approach. If the patient scores over a certain score, they are further evaluated by the PHQ-9 which asks questions in further detail and can assess the severity of depression.

PHQ-2

Over the past 2 weeks, how often have you been bothered by any of the following problems?	Not At All	Several Days	More Than Half the Days	Nearly Every Day
1. Little interest or pleasure in doing things	0	1	2	3
2. Feeling down, depressed or hopeless	0	1	2	3

If the patient scores 3 or more on PHQ-2, further assess the severity of depression using PHQ-9.

PHQ-9

Over the past 2 weeks, how often have you been bothered by any of the following problems?	Not At All	Several Days	More Than Half the Days	Nearly Every Day
1. Little interest or pleasure in doing things	0	1	2	3
2. Feeling down, depressed or hopeless	0	1	2	3
3. Trouble falling or staying asleep, or sleeping too much	0	1	2	3
4. Feeling tired or having little energy	0	1	2	3
5. Poor appetite or overeating	0	1	2	3
6. Feeling bad about yourself, or that you are a failure or have let yourself or your family down	0	1	2	3

7. Trouble concentrating on things	0	1	2	3
8. Moving or speaking so slowly that other people could have noticed? Or feeling the opposite- being fidgety or restless that you have been moving around a lot more than usual	0	1	2	3
9. Thoughts that you would be better off dead, or of hurting yourself in some way	0	1	2	3

Depression Severity:
0-4= None, 5-9= Mild, 10-14= Moderate, 15-19= Moderately Severe, 20-27= Severe

Case 2: Eating disorder

Candidate instructions

You are the foundation year doctor working in General Practice and have been asked to see Jenny a 19 years old who has presented to the GP surgery with weight loss. She is accompanied by her mother who is sitting outside in the waiting room as the patient has asked to see you alone. Please take a full history.

After 6 minutes the examiner will stop you and ask you to summarise back your findings, suggest your differential diagnoses and your initial management plan.

Examiner Instructions

Miss Jenkins is 19 years old has presented to the GP surgery accompanied by her mother who is sitting outside in the waiting room as the patient has asked to be seen alone.

The candidate, is acting as the foundation year doctor Doctor, and has been asked to take a history from the patient.

After 6 minutes please stop the candidate and ask them to present the case with their primary differential diagnoses. Following this ask them what their next steps regarding investigations and management will be.

If they ask, give them the examination findings below:
Examination findings: BMI 16.5. Observations are normal. All systemic examinations are normal. However she looks very thin.

Questions to ask if there is time:
What are the differences between anorexia nervosa and bulimia?

Actor Instructions

You are Miss Jenkins, a 19 years old who has presented to the GP surgery accompanied by your mother who is sitting outside in the waiting room, as you have asked to be seen alone.

ONLY OFFER INFORMATION IF SPECIFICALLY ASKED

You have come to see the doctor today as your mum has become concerned with regards to your weight. Your mum is concerned because you have lost approximately 2 stone in the past 3 months. However you feel fine and don't know why your mum is worried as you feel fat and feel like you need to lose weight.

You broke up with your boyfriend of 1 year approximately 4 months ago and was very upset over it. You had found out that he had cheated on you with a girl who you think is much skinnier and prettier than you, and think that he did that because you are fat. You therefore started going to the gym more often and now go at least 5-6 times per week. You also enjoy running and playing tennis and you try to do this as often as possible. You eat a healthy diet, but have recently cut out carbohydrates, dairy products and refined sugar as you felt they were making you put on weight. You have never binged or made yourself throw up. You do not take any medications or laxatives to help you lose weight.

You currently weigh 42kg and have a BMI of 16.5, and although you know this is lower than the healthy range you still feel like you need to lose weight. You are currently studying Law at Oxford University and you are due to sit your exams in the next two months. You have been finding it very difficult to juggle your university work with going to the gym, and have fallen behind with your work. You have been feeling more tired and sometimes find it difficult to concentrate.

You have also noticed that you haven't had your period for the past 2 months.

You do not smoke and you have cut out alcohol as it contains lots of calories. You do enjoy socialising but avoid it if it involves going out to eat. Your friends have noticed that you have become skinnier but you feel quite happy that people are noticing.

Your most recent visits home ended with you and your mum arguing over the dinner table as you refused to eat what she had cooked.

You had a happy childhood and was always very high achieving, however when you started secondary school you were bullied because of your weight. You have been feeling down because of the stress of exams but you have never had any thoughts of harming yourself.

You are usually fit and well with no other medical problems, and there is no history of eating disorders within the family.
If asked about your ideas, concerns and expectations please offer the information below
Your main concern is you want to be slim enough so that you can fit into a size 4 dress that you bought at the beginning of the month as motivation to lose weight.

Mark Scheme: Eating Disorder

	Achieved	Not Achieved
Introduces himself / herself		
Confirms patient details and purpose of consultation		
Established the main presenting complaint		
Elicits patient's thoughts about their weight		
Asks whether there was anything that triggered their recent weight loss		
Asks how much weight has been lost over what period of time		
Asks what their current diet and exercise regime is like		
Asks about taking any medications to help lose weight		
Asks about any binge eating or self-induced vomiting		
Asks about social and family life		
Asks about impact on education		
Asks about periods		
Asks about mood and screens for depression		
Asks about past psychiatric history		
Asks about past medical history, medications, allergies and family history		
Summarises findings concisely		
Able to provide appropriate differential diagnoses Anorexia nervosa		

Bulimia Depression		
Appropriate management plan & follow-up Cognitive behavioural therapy Family therapy Interpersonal therapy Referral to dietician Offers a review appointment to see how they are managing		
Acknowledges & addresses patient's ideas, concerns and expectations		
Gives patient opportunity to ask questions		
Examiner's Global Mark	/5	
Actor / Helper's Global Mark	/5	
Total Station Mark	/30	

Learning Points

- Anorexia nervosa is characterised by a distorted body image and excessive dieting that leads to severe weight loss with a pathological fear of becoming fat[1]. There is also disruption of the hypothalamus-pituitary axis, which can lead to amenorrhea in females and impotency in males.

- Bulimia nervosa is characterised by frequent episodes of binge-eating followed by self-induced vomiting to avoid weight gain[1].

- Treatments for anorexia nervosa and bulimia include psychological treatments such as cognitive behaviour therapy (CBT), interpersonal therapy (IPT) and family therapy.

References:
1. http://www.dsm5.org/Documents/Eating%20Disorders%20Fact%20Sheet.pdf

Case 3: Bipolar

Candidate Instructions

You are the foundation year doctor working in General Practice and have been asked to see Gemma a 24yr old woman, has presented to the GP surgery as her mother has become concerned by her behaviour. Please take a full history.

After 6 minutes the examiner will stop you and ask you to summarise back your findings, suggest your differential diagnoses and your initial management plan.

Examiner Instructions

Gemma a 24yr old woman, has presented to the GP surgery as her mother has become concerned by their behaviour.

The candidate, is acting as the foundation year doctor, and has been asked to take a history from the patient.

After 6 minutes please stop the candidate at and ask them to present the case with their primary differential diagnoses. Following this ask them what their next steps regarding investigations and management will be.

Questions to ask if there is time:
What is the treatment for Bipolar disorder and what are the side effects?

Actor's Instructions

When acting, try to appear hyperactive with fast speech and lots of hand gestures

You are Miss Green, a 24yr old woman, who has presented to the GP surgery as her mother has become concerned by their behaviour.

ONLY OFFER INFORMATION IF SPECIFICALLY ASKED

You are not sure why she is so worried, as you feel 'on top of the world' and have never felt better. In fact, you just bought a brand new car on your credit card despite not having a driving licence, and plan to travel across the world in it. Your mum has tried to dissuade you but you know that she is just being over-protective. Your current mood is a complete contrast to how you were feeling 6 months ago. Back then, you felt very low and spent most of your time sitting in your room watching TV. You stopped meeting up with friends, and felt tired and lethargic most of the time. You were working as an administration assistant in an office but unfortunately lost your job as you could not find the energy to leave the house in the morning.

About 2 weeks ago, you got another job, this time working in a coffee shop. However, since you started to feel much better, you have found it very difficult to concentrate on your daily tasks and frequently jump from one task to the next. This has been noticed by your employer who has issued you with a warning. You were initially worried about losing your job again, but realised that it might be a good thing as you will be quitting soon anyway to travel around the world in your car.

You don't smoke or drink alcohol, and you tend not to eat much during the day as you are so busy with your thoughts. You live at home with your parents and they have been worried for a long time about your mood. You are currently single.

If asked about your ideas, concerns and expectations please offer the information below

If the doctor asks you about what your thoughts are with regards to your behaviour, you mention that you don't know why everyone's so worried as you will become the most famous car driver in the world. Your mum has mentioned something about 'manic depression' which you would like to know more about. Ask questions regarding what treatment options are available.

Mark Scheme

	Achieved	Not Achieved
Introduces himself / herself		
Confirms patient details and purpose of consultation		
Established the main presenting complaint		
Asks about what concerns the patient's mother has		
Asks if the patient has the same concerns		
Asks about any grand or optimistic plans		
Asks about previous low mood, if she found little interest or pleasure in doing things, hopelessness		
Asks about impact of current mood on work life		
Asks about impact of current mood on social life		
Asks about eating and appetite, sleeping habits		
Assesses suicidal risk by asking specifically about thoughts of self harm		
Asks specifically about hearing or seeing things which aren't there		
Asks about past medical history, medications and allergies		
Asks about family history & social history including alcohol and smoking		
Summarises findings concisely		
Able to provide appropriate differential diagnoses Bipolar disorder Mania Psychosis		

Appropriate management plan & follow-up If patient is vulnerable or at harm to herself or to others consider admission to a psychiatric unit. Medical management - lithium Offers a review appointment to see how they are managing.		
Offers written information and helplines in case of emergency		
Acknowledges & addresses patient's ideas, concerns and expectations		
Gives patient opportunity to ask questions		
Examiner's Global Mark	/5	
Actor / Helper's Global Mark	/5	
Total Station Mark	/30	

Learning Points

- There are two types of bipolar disorder:
  - Type I - both depressive and manic symptoms develop at some point in the condition
  - Type II - patients develop hypomania

- The average length of an episode of mania is approximately four months, and an episode of depression lasts 6 months on average. However, both can be longer. Support will be delivered by the mental health team however the GP and practice have an important role in supporting the patient through both acute and stable periods.

- Treatment can be aimed at preventing episodes of mania or depression (mood-stabilisers, e.g. Lithium). Treatments can also be given only for when the episodes of depression or mania occur.

Chapter 12: Communication & Ethico legal

Case 1: Angry Patient

Candidate Instructions

You are the foundation year doctor working in General Practice and have been asked to see Jenn a 31 years old who has presented to the GP surgery. You can see from her notes that they came to see another GP in the practice, 3 days ago and was diagnosed with a viral URTI.

Take a full history and discuss your management plan with the patient and address her ideas, concerns and expectations

Examiner Instructions

Jenny a 31 years old has presented to the GP surgery. You can see from her notes that they came to see another GP in the practice, 3 days ago and was diagnosed with a viral URTI.

The candidate, is acting as the foundation year doctor, and has been asked to take a history from the patient.

After 6 minutes please stop the candidate and ask them to address the patients ideas, concerns and expectations and discuss your management plan.

If you feel the candidate is focusing too much on the clinical history- prompt them to move onto the social history.

Patient Instructions

You are Jenny a 31 years old, has presented to the GP surgery. You can see from her notes that they came to see another GP in the practice, 3 days ago and was diagnosed with a viral URTI.

ONLY OFFER INFORMATION IF SPECIFICALLY ASKED OR OPEN QUESTIONS ASKED

You are very worried about a cough which you have had for the past 5 days, and would like a chest x-ray. You came to see another Dr at the practice 3 days ago who told you it was a virus, and your symptoms since then have started to improve. You don't feel that the first doctor listened properly to you, and you felt like you were rushed out of the consultation before you could tell the doctor why you felt so worried. You dismiss the first consultation, telling the doctor that you thought his colleague was 'rubbish'.

Your cough started five days ago and is dry. You also had a runny nose and sore throat at the time the cough started, but both of those have resolved. Your cough is also improving. You have not had any of the following: Fevers, rigors, vomiting or problems with breathing currently or in the past.

You are worried about your cough as your father, a 62 year old heavy smoker, was diagnosed with lung cancer 2 weeks ago. As such, you are extremely worried about your symptoms as your father also had a cough prior to his diagnosis. He had seen his GP and was initially told that he had a viral infection, however he had also been coughing up blood and had lost 2 stone in weight in the past 6 months, despite having a normal appetite. His GP referred him urgently under the 2 week wait rule and imaging showed a suspicious mass in one of his lungs. He was then seen quickly by a specialist and he was confirmed to have lung cancer.

You have not been coughing up any blood, you have not had any weight loss and you are otherwise completely fit and well. You have not had any other symptoms except those listed above.

You live with your partner but your father lives alone since your mother passed away 5 years ago. Since then, you have noticed that your father's health has gradually deteriorated and you have had to take a lot of time off work to take him to various hospital appointments and look after him. You work as a lawyer and your company has not been very supportive recently, which has made you very stressed and upset.

You mention that have been taking your stress out on your partner who has tried to be supportive, and you have recently been having a lot of arguments.

If asked about your ideas, concerns and expectations please offer the information below

- **Ideas:** If you are asked whether you have had any thoughts or ideas about what your cough might be, shrug and say 'I don't know but I want you to do a chest x-ray so you can find out what it is'.
- **Concerns:** If you are asked what you are concerned about, or why you want an x-ray, say 'I'm just really worried about cancer'. Ask why the doctor isn't going to do a chest x-ray and begin to get angry and impatient, but calm down if you feel they are listening to your concerns and picking up on your verbal cues.
- **Expectations:** If you are asked what your expectations are, or you would like the doctor to do, say that you would like them to do a chest X-ray

If you feel that the doctor has elicited all of your concerns and worries, including those related to your personal life and work, and explains clearly without medical jargon why they feel your cough is a viral illness that doesn't need a chest x-ray, leave the consultation calmly when finished.

If you do not feel that the doctor has been empathic, or you do not feel they have explained why you do not need an x-ray, become angry and exasperated and walk out of the consultation

Mark Scheme: The Angry Patient

	Achieved	Not Achieved
Introduces himself / herself		
Confirms patient details and purpose of consultation		
Established the main presenting complaint and elicits brief history		
Asks about red flags – weight loss, change in appetite, haemoptysis, night sweats, persistent cough for >3weeks		
Remains neutral when the patient tells them that they thought their colleague was 'rubbish'		
Reassures patient that symptoms are due to a viral URTI		
Reassures patient that they do not need an x-ray and explains why		
Remains calm when patient becomes angry		
Picks up on verbal cues regarding work and home life and asks questions regarding this		
Asks specifically about support at home		
Elicits patient's thoughts or ideas as to what they think the cough might be		
Elicits the patient's concerns about the cough		
Elicits their expectations from this consultation		
Asks specifically why the patient is worried about cancer		
Listens empathically about father's condition		

Uses open questions throughout consultation and avoids using medical jargon		
Uses appropriate body language		
Comes up with a suitable management plan with patient, or safety nets		
Gives patient opportunity to ask questions		
Thanks patient		
Examiner's Global Mark	/5	
Actor / Helper's Global Mark	/5	
Total Station Mark	/30	

Learning Points

- Exploring the ideas, concerns and expectations allows you to fully understand why the patient may be angry or upset during the consultation. This may take time but this investment will be worth it in the long run. The patient is entitled to feel their experience was less satisfactory than they would have wished. Saying that you are sorry they feel this way is not an admission of guilt or bad practice.

- Verbal cues are easily missed- listening is key! Respond to these cues- the actors have been briefed so if they mention in passing that they are worried about something, explore those concerns.

- Using open questions allows the actor to tell you important bits of information that may otherwise have been missed, and can open up further areas of the consultation which can be explored.

Case 2: Breaking Bad News

Candidate's Instructions

William a 64 year old man has come in to the GP surgery to discuss his colonoscopy results. The results show there is a suspicious lesion and a biopsy confirms bowel cancer.

You are the foundation year doctor doctor in the GP and have been asked to discuss the results with the patient and suggest an appropriate management plan and address his ideas, concerns and expectations.

Examiner's Instructions

William a 64 year old man has come in to the GP surgery to discuss his colonoscopy results. The results show there is a suspicious lesion and a biopsy confirms bowel cancer. The patient is unaware of the results. He thinks he has been called in like last time to say the screening is normal.

The foundation year doctor doctor in the GP and have been asked to discuss the results with the patient and suggest an appropriate management plan and address his ideas, concerns and expectations.
As this is a communication station there is no need to stop the candidate at 6 minutes. Allow the candidate to start closing the consultation and give advice/arrange appropriate follow up.

Actor's Instructions

You are William a 64 year old man who has come in to the GP surgery to discuss his colonoscopy results.

This is your first colonoscopy after having your second routine screening FOB (Faecal occult blood. Which is a screening test that people aged 60-75 are offered every 2 years. A testing kit is received through the post).

The second time you did the FOB, you were called to have a colonoscopy. The reason for this was not communicated to you clearly, and you were not aware that the FOB was suspicious and that's why you had to have the colonoscopy. You have come alone and would not like anyone with you.

You have no expectation that it may be abnormal. Initially you are in disbelief and say the results are wrong and a mistake must've been made. Allow the candidate to break the news that the results are correct. At this point you are distraught when you find out. You start to cry and think that you are going to die.

Your brother died of colorectal cancer a year ago. You have a good support network including 2 adult children and your wife.

If the candidate says "I understand how you're feeling/ what you're going through", immediately ask "Have you been through this? Do you have bowel cancer? How can you understand what I'm going through?"

If candidate uses technical terms such as 'lesion' or alarming words 'tumour' appear worried/surprised/confused.

If patient uses silence after breaking the bad news, and doesn't interrupt you, you should ask a question e.g. "what happens next?"

If asked about your ideas, concerns and expectations please offer the information below
You don't know where to start, you are worried about what will happen to your wife if you weren't around anymore. You are unable to process this all so quickly.

Mark Scheme: Breaking Bad News

Task:	Achieved	Not Achieved
Introduces himself / herself		
Confirms patient details and purpose of consultation		
Established the main reason for attendance and elicits brief history		
Asks if anyone has come with them or if they would like someone present		
Finds out what patient's understanding is thus far		
Gives a warning shot		
Gives clear information regarding the results - uses the word 'cancer'		
Avoids use of jargon		
Ensures patient understands the importance of the information		
Listens empathically about brother's condition		
Uses silence as a tool, before continuing with consultation		
Uses appropriate body language		
Ensures patient absorbs information		
Explains what will happen next		
Comes up with a suitable management plan with patient - including follow up appointment		
Summarises consultation & actions from here on		
Offers additional written material		

Acknowledges & addresses patient's ideas, concerns and expectations		
Gives patient opportunity to ask questions		
Thanks patient		
Examiner's Global Mark	/5	
Actor / Helper's Global Mark	/5	
Total Station Mark	/30	

Learning Points

- Ensure you have prepared the environment and settings. Quiet room, layout of chairs/desk. Always ask if they would like someone with them.

- Don't be afraid to use silence as a tool, allow the patient to lead the consultation, they will ask when they're ready

- The most important thing is to ensure the patient feels supported by you and your team. Make a follow up appointment for them to come back with written questions. "We will do this together step by step". "This must be a lot to take in, I will provide you with some leaflets for you to look through in your own time, and we can discuss things you don't understand when I see you next" "Please do contact me if you have any concerns or questions"

Case 3: Gillick Competence & Confidentiality

Candidate's Instructions

You are the foundation year doctor working in General Practice and have been asked to see Ella a 14 year old girl has presented to the GP surgery to discuss contraception with you.

Take a full history and discuss your management plan with the patient and address her ideas, concerns and expectations. The examiner will assess your knowledge of confidentiality and gillick competence.

Examiner's Instructions

Ella a 14 year old girl has presented to the GP surgery to discuss contraception with you.

The candidate, is acting as the foundation year doctor and has been asked to take a history from the patient.

After 6 minutes please stop the candidate at whatever stage they are and ask them to discuss their next steps regarding management and address patients ideas, concerns and expectations.

Additional questions:

- What are the requirements of the fraser guidelines?
- Who would you like to discuss this with?
- Under what age would it be illegal for a person to have intercourse?
- Can the GP prescribe the OCP to this patient without her parents' consent?
- How would you assess for competency?

Actor's Instructions

Ella a 14 year old girl has presented to the GP surgery to discuss contraception with you.

ONLY OFFER INFORMATION IF SPECIFICALLY ASKED

You are in a relationship with a 15 year old boy. You have started having sexual intercourse over the last 2 months. Up until now you have been using condoms but would like to switch to the oral contraceptive pill (OCP) as you feel it would be more reliable. Your friend is on the OCP and she has advised that you also start it. You have consented to sexual intercourse and your boyfriend has never forced you to have sexual intercourse.

You would not like to tell your parents as you don't want them to know that you are having sexual intercourse. You feel they would get angry about having sexual intercourse at this age.

You and your boyfriend have been to a sexual health clinic to get yourselves checked out for previous sexually transmitted infections and both of you have been cleared. You have never fallen pregnant either. Your main reason for wanting the OCP is so that you don't have to rely on condoms. You feel that now that your relationship is stable and believe it is a long term relationship, you would like to switch to the OCP.

You are currently studying for you GCSEs and live with your parents and brother. You are an organized person and will remember to take the pill at the same time every day. There is no family history of blood clots in the family and you are otherwise fit and well. Your BMI is 21, you don't smoke nor do you drink alcohol. You have never taken any illicit drugs.

Even if the doctor doesn't prescribe you the OCP you will continue to have intercourse. You do not want any other form of contraception like the coil or implant as you do not like the idea of something foreign being in your body.

If asked about your ideas, concerns and expectations please offer the information below

You are concerned about falling pregnant as you are young and feel that having a baby would stop you from progressing in your education.

Mark Scheme: Gillick Competence & Confidentiality

Task:	Achieved	Not Achieved
Introduces himself / herself		
Confirms patient details and purpose of consultation		
Established the main reason for attendance		
Establishes age of patient and her boyfriend		
Asks if she is consenting to sexual intercourse and whether she has ever felt forced to have intercourse or anything sexual in origin with anyone		
Asks if she has ever fallen pregnant?		
Has she or her partner had any sexually transmitted diseases?		
Current mode of contraception?		
Are her parents aware? Why has she not told her parents?		
Can she be convinced to tell her parents?		
Does she understand the professional advice?		
Establishes that she is likely to continue having sexual intercourse with her boyfriend regardless of the doctor providing the pill		
Offers to discuss other forms of contraception		
Non judgmental approach		
Comes up with a suitable management plan with patient - including follow up appointment		

Summarises consultation & actions from here on		
Offers additional written material		
Acknowledges & addresses patient's ideas, concerns and expectations		
Gives patient opportunity to ask questions		
Answers examiners questions appropriately		
Examiner's Global Mark	/5	
Actor / Helper's Global Mark	/5	
Total Station Mark	/30	

Learning Points

- **Fraser guidelines:** With regards to the **provision of contraceptives** to patients under 16 years of age the Fraser Guidelines state that all the following requirements should be fulfilled:

  - the young person understands the professional's advice
  - the young person cannot be persuaded to inform their parents
  - the young person is likely to begin, or to continue having, sexual intercourse with or without contraceptive treatment
  - unless the young person receives contraceptive treatment, their physical or mental health, or both, are likely to suffer
  - the young person's best interests require them to receive contraceptive advice or treatment with or without parental consent

- **Gillick competence**
  - A term used in medical law to decide whether a child (16 years or younger) is able to consent to his or her own medical treatment, without the need for parental permission or knowledge

- The most important information to establish is whether there are any safeguarding issues here. If you felt that there were, you would escalate your concerns to your supervisor.

References

1. British Thoracic Society and Scottish Intercollegiate Guidelines Network. *British Guideline for the management of asthma.* 2014
2. NICE guideline (NG12). *Suspected cancer: recognition and referral.* June 2015
3. NICE pathways. *Crohns disease.* May 2016
4. NICE pathways. *Ulcerative colitis.* May 2016
5. NICE guidelines (NG3). *Diabetes in pregnancy: management from preconception to the postnatal period.* August 2015.
6. US Department Of Health And Human Services Centers For Disease Control And Prevention. *A guide to taking a sexual history.* 2005
7. NICE Clinical Guideline [CG156]. *Fertility Problems: Assessment and treatment.* February 2015
8. Pfizer. *Instructions for Patient Health Questionnaire (PHQ) and GAD-7 Measures. Patient Health Questionnaire (PHQ) Screeners.* 1999
9. NICE Clinical guideline (CG9). *Eating disorders in over 8s: management.* January 2004
10. NICE Local Government briefing (LGB17). *Contraceptive services.* March 2014

Printed in Great Britain
by Amazon